WITHDRAWN

STACKS

W9-BUC-002

HOW
NUTRITION
WORKS

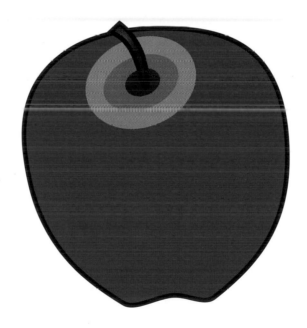

HOW NUTRITION WORKS DESCRIBES NUTRITIONAL NEEDS IN GENERAL AND DISCUSSES THE EFFECTS OF MINERAL AND VITAMIN DEFICIENCIES ON THE HUMAN BODY. IT TRIES TO MAKE YOU A SMARTER CONSUMER OF HEALTH SERVICES AND PRODUCTS, BUT IT DOES NOT OFFER MEDICAL ADVICE AND IS NOT A SUBSTITUTE FOR MEDICAL CARE OR SUPERVISION. CONSULT A PHYSICIAN ABOUT ALL YOUR SPECIFIC HEALTH CONCERNS.

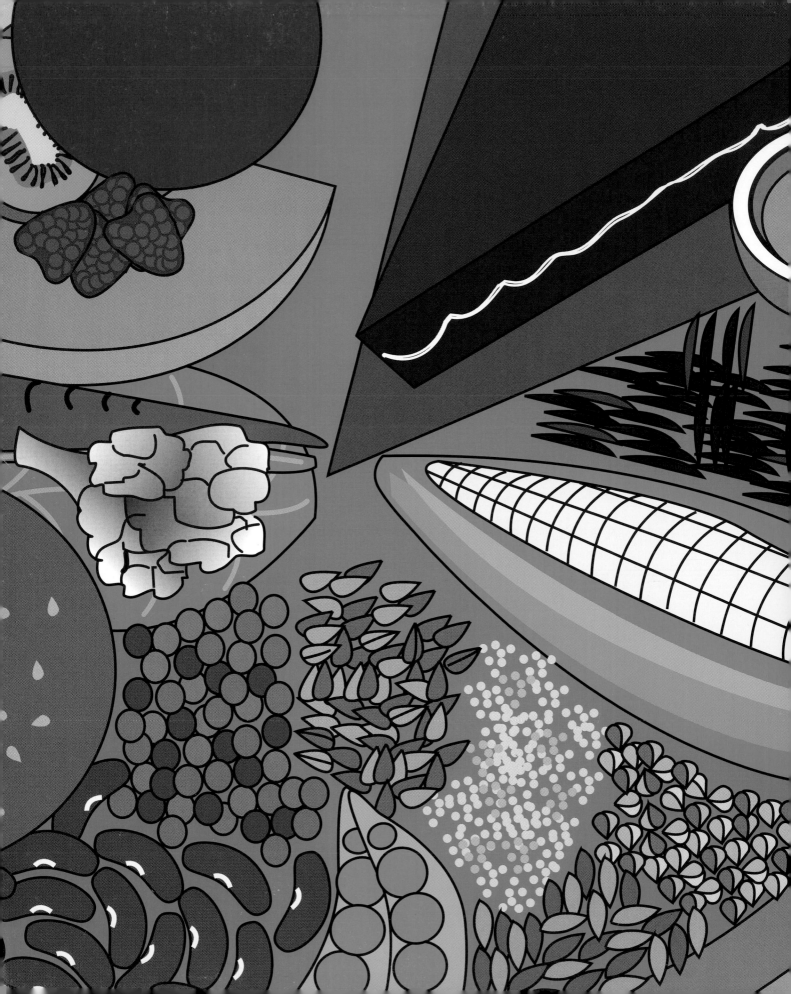

HOW
NUTRITION
WORKS

KRISTINE M. NAPIER, M.P.H., R.D.

Illustrated by
DEBRA MUROV

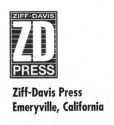

Ziff-Davis Press
Emeryville, California

Development Editor	Mary Johnson
Copy Editor	Kelly Green
Technical Reviewer	Nancy Gustafson
Project Coordinator	Barbara Dahl
Proofreader	Carol Burbo
Cover Illustration	Debra Murov and Regan Honda
Cover Design	Regan Honda
Book Design	Carrie English
Technical Illustration	Debra Murov
Word Processing	Howard Blechman
Page Layout	Tony Jonick and M.D. Barrera
Indexer	Valerie Robbins

Ziff-Davis Press books are produced on a Macintosh computer system with the following applications: FrameMaker®, Microsoft® Word, QuarkXPress®, Adobe Illustrator®, Adobe Photoshop®, Adobe Streamline™, MacLink®*Plus*, Aldus® FreeHand™, Collage Plus™.

If you have comments or questions or would like to receive a free catalog, call or write:
Ziff-Davis Press
5903 Christie Avenue
Emeryville, CA 94608
1-800-688-0448

Copyright © 1995 by Kristine Napier. All rights reserved.
PART OF A CONTINUING SERIES

Ziff-Davis Press and ZD Press are trademarks of Ziff Communications Company.

All other product names and services identified throughout this book are trademarks or registered trademarks of their respective companies. They are used throughout this book in editorial fashion only and for the benefit of such companies. No such uses, or the use of any trade name, is intended to convey endorsement or other affiliation with the book.

No part of this publication may be reproduced in any form, or stored in a database or retrieval system, or transmitted or distributed in any form by any means, electronic, mechanical photocopying, recording, or otherwise, without the prior written permission of Ziff-Davis Press, except as permitted by the Copyright Act of 1976.

THE INFORMATION AND MATERIAL CONTAINED IN THIS BOOK ARE PROVIDED "AS IS," WITHOUT WARRANTY OF ANY KIND, EXPRESS OR IMPLIED, INCLUDING WITHOUT LIMITATION ANY WARRANTY CONCERNING THE ACCURACY, ADEQUACY, OR COMPLETENESS OF SUCH INFORMATION OR MATERIAL OR THE RESULTS TO BE OBTAINED FROM USING SUCH INFORMATION OR MATERIAL. NEITHER ZIFF-DAVIS PRESS NOR THE AUTHOR SHALL BE RESPONSIBLE FOR ANY CLAIMS ATTRIBUTABLE TO ERRORS, OMISSIONS, OR OTHER INACCURACIES IN THE INFORMATION OR MATERIAL CONTAINED IN THIS BOOK, AND IN NO EVENT SHALL ZIFF-DAVIS PRESS OR THE AUTHOR BE LIABLE FOR DIRECT, INDIRECT, SPECIAL, INCIDENTAL, OR CONSEQUENTIAL DAMAGES ARISING OUT OF THE USE OF SUCH INFORMATION OR MATERIAL.

ISBN 1-56276-254-0

Manufactured in the United States of America
⊕ This book is printed on paper that contains 50% total recycled fiber of which 20% is de-inked postconsumer fiber.
10 9 8 7 6 5 4 3 2 1

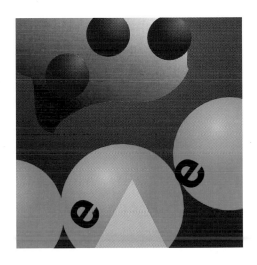

This book is dedicated to
Dr. Eric Mood, one of my
Yale professors, and to
Dr. Elizabeth Whelan, my
mentor, two people who have
helped me see that no one
topic can be considered in a
vacuum, and that keeping a
global perspective is essential
to all we encounter in life.

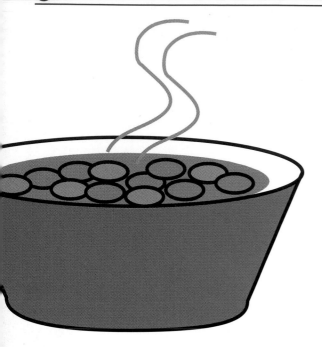

Introduction.................. xi

Macronutrients: More Than Calories

1

Chapter 1
Carbohydrates: High-Octane
Fuel for Working Bodies 4

Chapter 2
Protein: Brain, Growth,
Healing…and Living
Power 14

Chapter 3
Fat: Both Friend and Foe.... 26

Chapter 4
Balancing Macronutrients for
Awesome Health 34

Micronutrients: The Finer Details to Greater Health

44

Chapter 5
Fat-Soluble Vitamins: They
Stick to Your Ribs 48

Chapter 6
Water-Soluble Vitamins 56

Chapter 7
Vitamins as Antioxidants:
Radical Protection.......... 64

Chapter 8
Minerals: Lending Strength
and Glow to Good Health... 70

Chapter 9
Calcium: More Than Strong
Bones 80

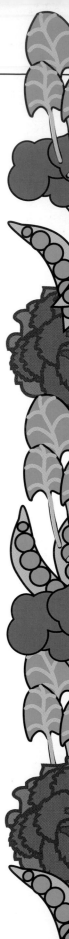
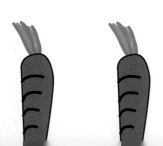
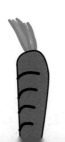
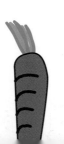
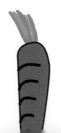
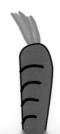
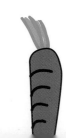

PART 3

How to Win Your Nutrition Battles

86

Chapter 10
Iron: How to Prevent the Most Common Nutritional Deficiency 90

Chapter 11
Nutrient Density: More Nutrition per Calorie 98

Chapter 12
How to Devise a Low-Fat Diet—and Stick to It 104

Chapter 13
How to Eat to Lower Cholesterol: Fact and Fad .. 112

Chapter 14
Re-salt Your Diet to Control Blood Pressure 124

Chapter 15
How to Get Enough Fiber to Fight Disease 132

Chapter 16
How to Stop Dieting and Be Trim 140

Chapter 17
How to Fight Cancer with a Healthy Diet 146

Chapter 18
You Still Have Questions... 154

Index 163

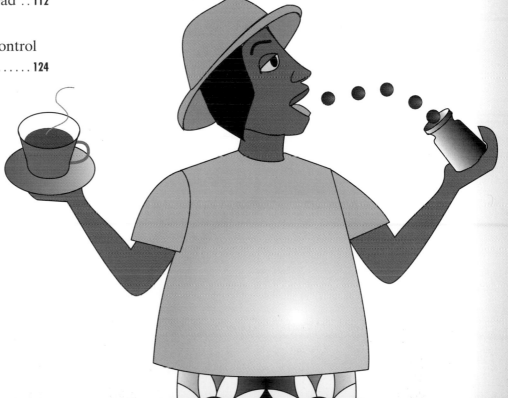

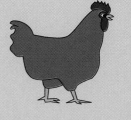

I am very grateful to the many people at Ziff-Davis Press who helped conceptualize this book, shape its development, and see it to completion: Cindy Hudson, president of Ziff-Davis Press, who encouraged me initially; Eric Stone, acquisitions editor, who was exceptionally helpful and attuned to the finest details; and to Mary Johnson, development editor, whose heartfelt enthusiasm, encouragement, and endless font of new ideas kept me on track. And, last, but not least, to the people at Ziff-Davis responsible for the tiniest and most important details of putting a book together: Kelly Green, copy editor, and Barbara Dahl, project editor.

My heartfelt thanks to the artist, Debra Murov, and her extraordinary artistic ability for turning my pencil scratches into lucid works of art.

My love and appreciation to my husband, Jim, and my children, Susie and Jim, for their patience, sense of humor, fresh perspective, and loving support.

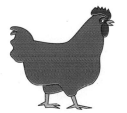 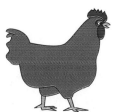 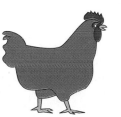 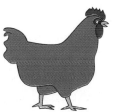

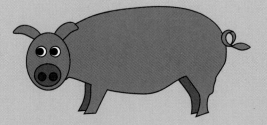

Having trouble keeping up with the latest nutrition news? Do you find yourself shunning one food for another as you hear that one food is bad and another is good? Are you forever trying to cram more bottles of supplements into your medicine cabinet as you read that one more vitamin, mineral, or other food substance is good for your health? And are you left totally confused about what to actually *eat?* Then this book about nutrition is for you.

This book will bring you up to date on the latest nutrition information and then will show you how to fashion an eating plan from real food that will help you trim down to a healthy weight (without dieting), maximize your energy, fight off diseases such as osteoporosis and heart disease, and help you perform better athletically.

The body is an amazingly intricate machine that craves just the right fuel mix to function optimally. But it's a rare American who eats this health-sustaining fuel mix. Although your body doesn't sputter to a stop as would a lawn mower that was fed the wrong mixture of oil and gas, over the long run you might find yourself feeling tired, sluggish, and just not up to par—but not really able to put your finger on why you don't feel 100%.

Believe it or not, millions of health-conscious Americans in this land of plenty are deficient in one or more essential nutrients, most without knowing it. The majority of American women don't get enough calcium, which places them at risk of osteoporosis and its life-changing debilities. Men and women aren't getting enough of several B vitamins, which increases their risk of heart disease and cancer, among other things. It's the rare American who gets enough of all essential minerals, which work in countless ways to keep the machinery of our bodies functioning optimally. At the same time, the majority of Americans eat far too much fat—especially saturated fat—which increases their risk for many maladies—cancer, heart disease, and obesity among them.

Nature has an incredible ability to pack into the healthiest foods many vitamins, minerals, and other substances we need for good health. Some vegetables, for example, are loaded with fiber and several essential vitamins and minerals and are nearly devoid of fat (and saturated fat). The same is true for fruits, legumes, and whole grains. At the same time, highly refined foods that are high in fat and calories come up close to empty on essential nutrients.

Read on to see why your body needs so many essential substances, why one can't substitute for another, and how to craft a diet that you thoroughly enjoy and that's right for your body's machinery.

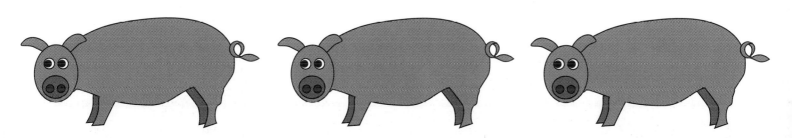

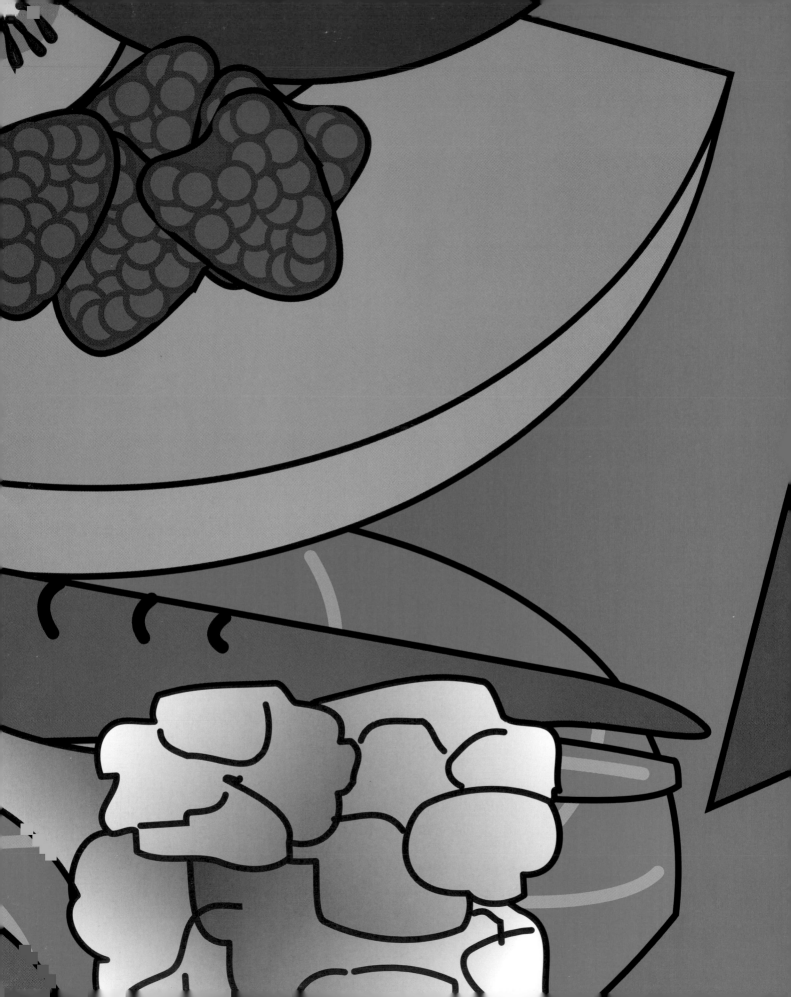

1

MACRONUTRIENTS: MORE THAN CALORIES

CONTENTS

Chapter 1   Carbohydrates: High-Octane Fuel
for Working Bodies
4

Chapter 2   Protein: Brain, Growth, Healing . . .
and Living Power
14

Chapter 3   Fat: Both Friend and Foe
26

Chapter 4   Balancing Macronutrients for
Awesome Health
34

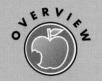

OVERVIEW

I F YOU'RE LIKE most Americans, you're concerned about your weight and you try to balance the number of calories you take in with the number you expend each day. And, if you're that typical American, you sometimes skip healthy food like fruits, vegetables, and milk so that you can fit in chips, candy bars, soda pop, and other favorite foods. But is it enough just to get the right *number* of calories?

Consider this analogy. If your lawn mower runs out of gas, can you put in just any mixture of gas and oil? Clearly not. But, unfortunately, the consequences of refueling the body with the wrong mix of calorie-containing nutrients aren't as obvious. While a lawn mower stutters to an immediate stop with the wrong type of fuel, bodies may run for many years without any obvious sign of malfunction. People who chronically eat the wrong mix of food may feel tired or just not up to par but never connect this to eating poorly. And deep within, diseases such as cancer, heart disease, and osteoporosis may be developing. The human body is indeed an intricate machine that craves the right mix of fuel to make it run smoothly.

Three types of nutrients, called macronutrients, supply the body with the energy it needs to keep going: carbohydrates, protein, and fat. To create just the right fuel mix, you have to fashion a diet of just the right percentages of these three macronutrients. In the following chapters, we'll translate the percentages into real terms: shopping carts and plates of food.

When you eat food that gives you the right mix of macronutrients, you automatically accrue an additional benefit: You stand an excellent chance of getting all the micronutrients your body needs to function well (see Part 2 for more information on micronutrients).

Read on to learn why the body needs each of these calorie-supplying nutrients, including fat, and then how to devise an eating plan that gives you just the right mix.

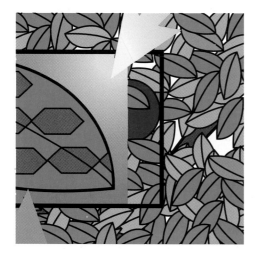

Carbohydrates: High-Octane Fuel for Working Bodies

REMEMBER THE DAYS when people watching their weight shunned bread, potatoes, pasta, or other carbohydrate-rich foods? The only carbohydrate calories on a diet plate came from a sprig of parsley, or maybe a canned peach half.

Today, fortunately, carbohydrates are in the health spotlight. Without a doubt, they're the highest quality fuel—the highest octane available—for working, growing bodies. When chosen properly, foods rich in carbohydrates are also rich in vitamins and minerals essential to great health. And woven into the complex carbohydrate bundle is dietary fiber, another essential thread of good health.

More good news: The best carbohydrates are almost fat free. Also, excess carbohydrate calories aren't as likely to turn into body fat. Although it's not a good idea to make a habit of eating excess calories, if you do, fewer extra carbohydrate calories are stored as body fat. That's because as much as 25% of excess carbohydrate calories are burned up as the "cost" of turning them into and storing them as fat. So, if you eat 100 extra carbohydrate calories on any given day, just 75 of these calories are tucked away as fat. In contrast, the cost of storing extra fat calories is just 3%, which means 97 of every 100 fat calories are stored as fat.

You may know carbohydrates by other names: starch, sugar, or glucose. Sugar is the common word for carbohydrates; starch and glucose are two types of sugar, or carbohydrate. Or you may have heard the terms *complex* and *simple* carbohydrates, which are different types of carbohydrates.

Glucose is one of the simplest sugars found in food, and it is the form of sugar to which all other types of sugar are eventually converted in the body. It's also the form of sugar carried in the bloodstream as the ultimate energy source that jump-starts cells, keeps us thinking clearly, and gives muscles fuel to perform. Fructose and galactose are other simple sugars found in foods such as fruit. All simple sugars are called monosaccharides—*mono* meaning *one* and *saccharide* meaning *sugar*.

Next on the carbohydrate ladder are the disaccharides, where *di* stands for *two*. Disaccharides are two simple sugars hooked together. Sucrose, the official chemical name for table sugar, is one example of a disaccharide.

At the top of the heap are the polysaccharides, or substances with many single sugars joined together. Rice, wheat, and soybeans are just some of the many foods containing polysaccharides, which are also called starch. That's why such foods are called starches.

But how do the terms *simple* and *complex* carbohydrates come into play? This time, let's start at the top and work down. Complex carbohydrate foods are made up primarily of polysaccharides. These foods aren't the most complex just in terms of how they are formed, but also because wrapped into their elaborate packages are lots of vitamins, minerals, sometimes protein (for example, the complex-carbohydrate foods lentils and split peas are high in protein), and fiber—and many health benefits. When we eat starchy foods, we benefit from the entire nutritional package, not just the polysaccharides.

Simple carbohydrates are foods containing mono- or disaccharides. Also called sweets, they include such favorite treats as honey, syrup, candy, desserts, soda pop, and sweetened cereals. We know that complex carbohydrates are by far the best choice; but are sugary foods, or simple carbohydrates, *bad*, as you may have read? Is sugar really responsible for heart disease, cancer, diabetes, and hyperactivity? Probably not, say leading experts convened by the U.S. Food and Drug Administration as the Sugar Task Force. But there are still plenty of reasons to keep your intake of pure simple sugars in check.

All carbohydrates supply 4 calories per gram. A medium apple, for example, contains about 20 grams of carbohydrate and has 80 calories. Many foods, like the apple, contain water and other substances, so you can't weigh foods to determine their carbohydrate content. The apple itself, for example, weighs about 138 grams.

Most simple carbohydrates are also called empty calorie foods because they have very few, if any, nutrients other than calories. (Yes, that's true even for honey.) This is because the sugars are *refined*, or unwrapped from that complex carbohydrate package. Put another way, the sugar is stripped from its source, leaving behind the vitamins, minerals, and fiber.

Corn syrup, for example, is refined from corn. Let's compare an equal number of calories supplied by corn syrup and corn kernels. One-half cup of corn kernels has about 65 calories and, in addition to its carbohydrates, is a good source of dietary fiber, vitamin A, folate and other B vitamins, and minerals such as magnesium, phosphorus, and potassium. About 60 calories of corn syrup (even the dark variety) has no fiber and barely discernible traces of vitamins and minerals. In addition, less than 1% of corn syrup is complex carbohydrate, where 80% of corn kernal carbohydrate is complex.

Eating too many simple carbohydrates, or refined sugars, upsets your nutrition profile for at least three reasons. Eating such foods uses up some of your daily calorie budget, leaving fewer calories for complex carbohydrates (and essential nutrients).

Also, foods that satisfy your sweet tooth are frequently laced with fat. A small chocolate candy bar with nuts, for example, has just 238 calories, but nearly 18 grams of fat. Finally, simple carbohydrates fall very short on fiber.

But what about fruits? Because most fruits contain simple sugars and not complex carbohydrates, are they a poor nutritional choice? Absolutely not! Fruits have plenty of vitamins, minerals, and fiber. And because many are high in water, they also help you fill up on relatively few calories. Think of fruit as simple sugars wrapped into a complex nutritional package.

Carbohydrates should make up the bulk of your daily eating plan. At least 60% of your daily calories should come from carbohydrates, and 4 of every 5 carbohydrate calories (or 80%) should be complex. Unfortunately, Americans have some work to do to achieve this healthy goal.

The average American consumes only 40% to 50% of calories as carbohydrates, and only about half of that as fruits, grains, vegetables, and other high-quality or complex carbohydrates. Currently, Americans eat the other half as table sugar and high-fructose corn syrup, which is used to sweeten such items as soda pop, cereals, prepared spaghetti sauces, fruit juices, and yogurts. That means Americans eat the equivalent of more than 16 teaspoons of sugar each day, or 60 pounds of table sugar and 50 pounds of corn syrup each year. In contrast, 100 years ago the average American consumed just 4 pounds of table sugar in an entire year. People in developing countries, whose dietary staples are such foods as rice and beans, do a much better job of consuming complex carbohydrates than do Americans.

Begin to think of complex carbohydrates as your dietary staple. Aim for doubling up on foods like grains, pastas, vegetables, and fruits at mealtime, filling two-thirds of your plate with these complex nutrition packages.

Most of Your Carbohydrates Should Be Complex

It's time for an adventure in eating! At least 80% of your carbohydrate intake should be nutritionally rich complex carbohydrates. Only 20% of a day's carbohydrate calories should come from refined, or simple, carbohydrates. Toward the goal of eating 60% of your daily calories as carbohydrates, try some of the foods described here.

Complex carbohydrates   Daily choose some from each category:

Cereal grains. Included among the common varieties are wheat, rye, rice, corn, and oats; among the not-so-common are barley, quinoa, and millet. Try them as the whole grain, as a side dish, or in a casserole, or try breads and bagels made from their flours.

Legumes. Try all of these nutrient-packed carbs: black beans, chick peas, kidney beans, brown and red lentils, soybeans (as tofu or the bean), and peanuts.

Vegetables. Daily get some of each type: green leafy (romaine lettuce, spinach), yellow/red (carrots, winter squash), and cruciferous (broccoli, cauliflower, brussel sprouts).

Fruits. Try berries and bananas, melons and more: Go for 2–3 types daily.

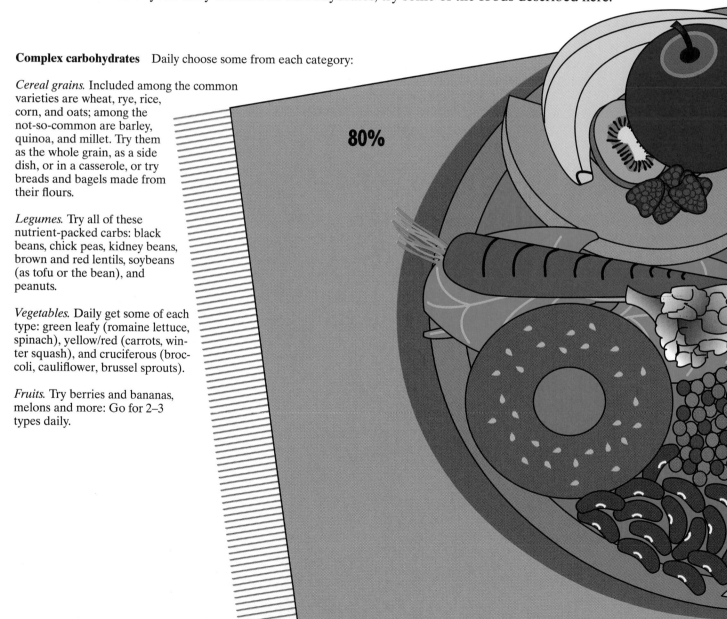

80%

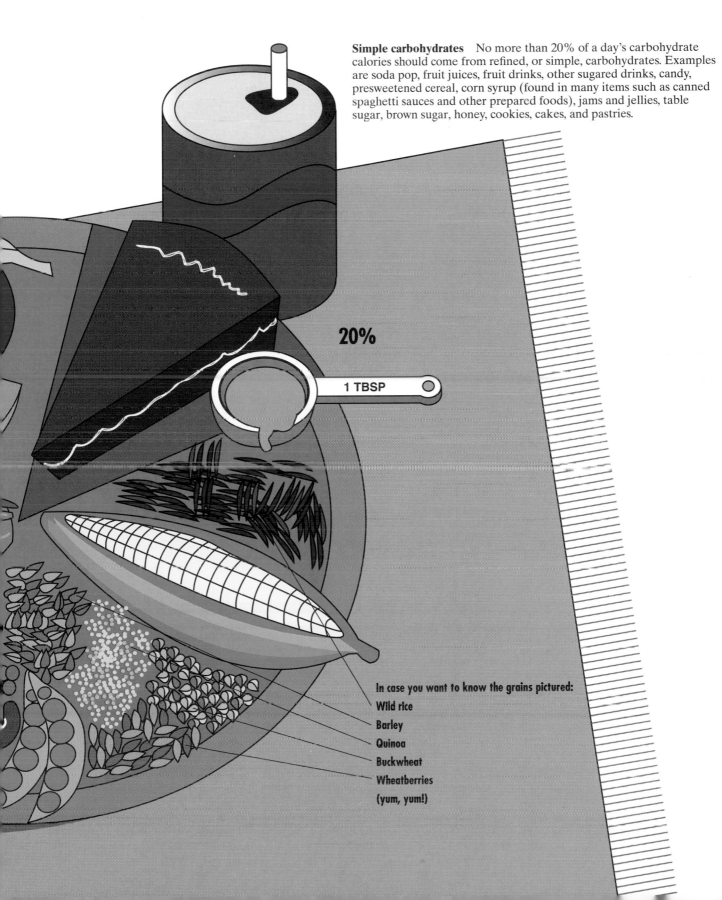

Simple carbohydrates No more than 20% of a day's carbohydrate calories should come from refined, or simple, carbohydrates. Examples are soda pop, fruit juices, fruit drinks, other sugared drinks, candy, presweetened cereal, corn syrup (found in many items such as canned spaghetti sauces and other prepared foods), jams and jellies, table sugar, brown sugar, honey, cookies, cakes, and pastries.

20%

1 TBSP

In case you want to know the grains pictured:

Wild rice

Barley

Quinoa

Buckwheat

Wheatberries

(yum, yum!)

How Nature Makes Carbohydrates

Carbohydrates are truly a natural wonder. Green plants transform water in soil and carbon dioxide in the air, with the aid of the sun's energy, into chemical energy. That chemical energy takes the form of sugar, or carbohydrate, as it's more formally called.

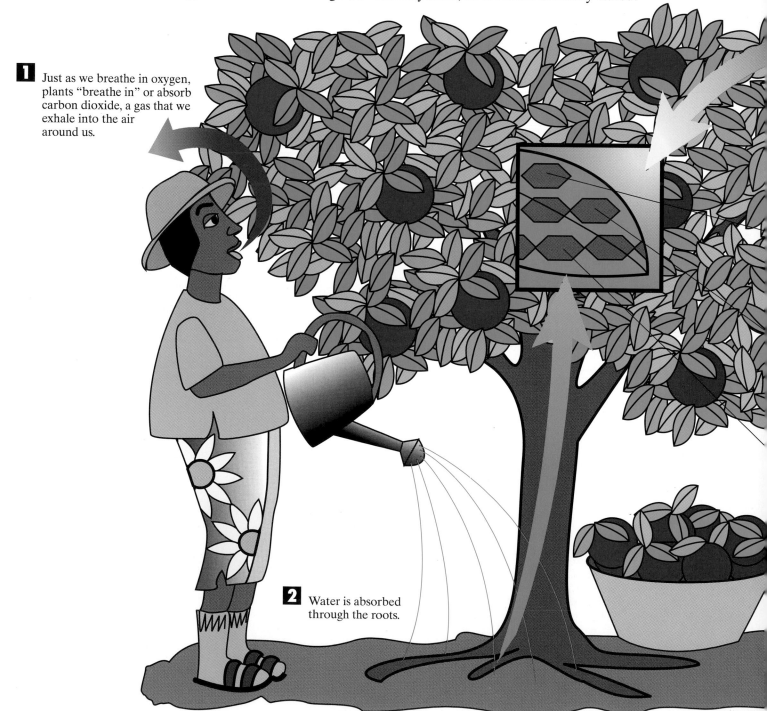

1 Just as we breathe in oxygen, plants "breathe in" or absorb carbon dioxide, a gas that we exhale into the air around us.

2 Water is absorbed through the roots.

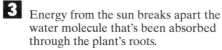

3 Energy from the sun breaks apart the water molecule that's been absorbed through the plant's roots.

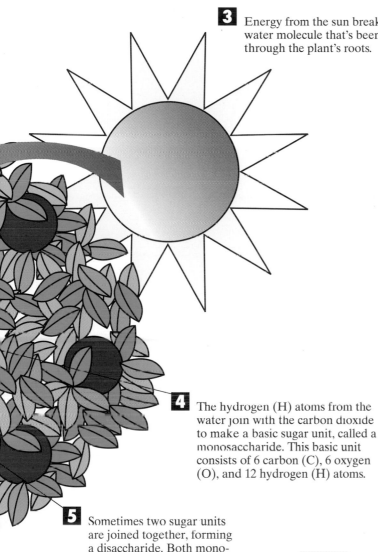

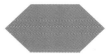

Monosaccharides, or one-sugar units, are galactose (found in milk sugar), glucose (found in fruits, vegetables, and honey), and fructose (found in fruits, artichokes, and honey).

4 The hydrogen (H) atoms from the water join with the carbon dioxide to make a basic sugar unit, called a monosaccharide. This basic unit consists of 6 carbon (C), 6 oxygen (O), and 12 hydrogen (H) atoms.

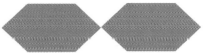

Disaccharides include maltose, two units of glucose joined together (abundant in germinated grains); sucrose, a unit of fructose and one of glucose (abundant in sugar beets and the sap of sugar maples); and lactose, glucose plus galactose (found in milk).

5 Sometimes two sugar units are joined together, forming a disaccharide. Both mono- and disaccharides dissolve in the watery juices of plants, which facilitates their transport from one part of the plant to another.

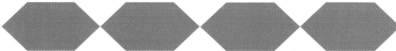

6 Some mono- and disaccharides are tucked away in the juice for later uses, but the majority joins together to form large units called polysaccharides.

Polysaccharides consist of hundreds to thousands of simple sugar units joined together. Plants store carbohydrates as starch, as cellulose, and as other fibrous carbohydrates. Both starch and cellulose are composed of hundreds of glucose units joined together, but in different configurations. People store carbohydrates as glycogen, another polysaccharide composed of hundreds of glucose units.

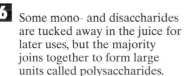

How the Body Burns Carbohydrates as Fuel

All dietary carbohydrates are broken up by the body into their simplest sugars and eventually converted to glucose, which supplies energy to every cell in the body. Although most tissues throughout the body can use protein and fat as fuel (though much less efficiently), the brain, nervous tissue, lungs, and hemoglobin (iron-carrying portion of red blood cells) can use only glucose. Carbohydrates are the highest-octane and most efficient fuel for growing and working bodies.

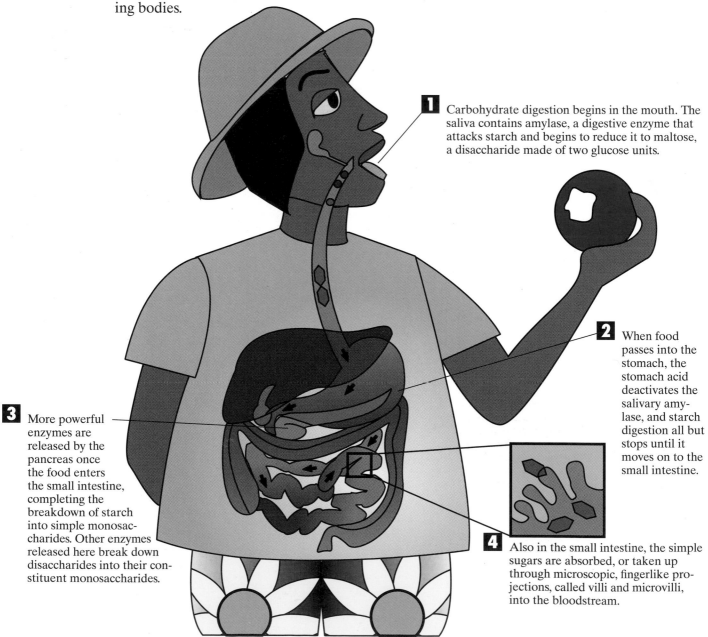

1 Carbohydrate digestion begins in the mouth. The saliva contains amylase, a digestive enzyme that attacks starch and begins to reduce it to maltose, a disaccharide made of two glucose units.

2 When food passes into the stomach, the stomach acid deactivates the salivary amylase, and starch digestion all but stops until it moves on to the small intestine.

3 More powerful enzymes are released by the pancreas once the food enters the small intestine, completing the breakdown of starch into simple monosaccharides. Other enzymes released here break down disaccharides into their constituent monosaccharides.

4 Also in the small intestine, the simple sugars are absorbed, or taken up through microscopic, fingerlike projections, called villi and microvilli, into the bloodstream.

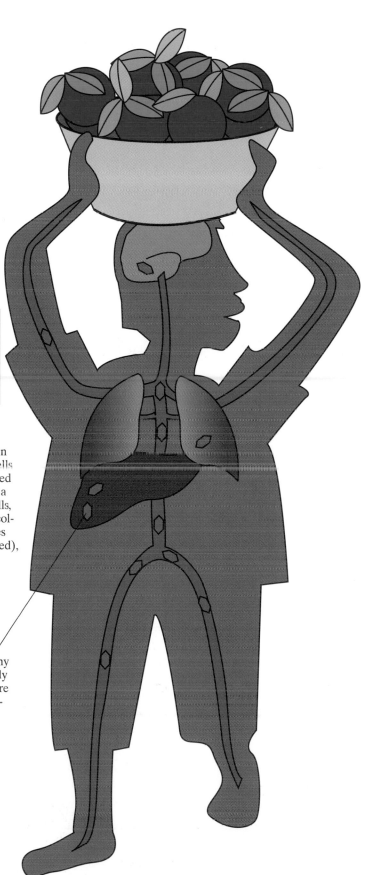

5 Once in the bloodstream, the fate of glucose molecules depends on the body's needs. Glucose continuously feeds the brain and other nervous tissues, lungs, and hemoglobin, as these tissues and cells cannot function without it. Unlike other body tissues, they cannot use any other type of fuel. Largely because of this, the body must maintain a certain level of blood sugar.

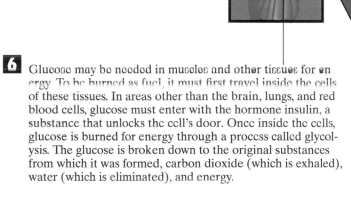

6 Glucose may be needed in muscles and other tissues for energy. To be burned as fuel, it must first travel inside the cells of these tissues. In areas other than the brain, lungs, and red blood cells, glucose must enter with the hormone insulin, a substance that unlocks the cell's door. Once inside the cells, glucose is burned for energy through a process called glycolysis. The glucose is broken down to the original substances from which it was formed, carbon dioxide (which is exhaled), water (which is eliminated), and energy.

7 When there is too much glucose in the bloodstream, it is carried to the liver, where it is converted to glycogen (many units of glucose hooked together) and stored. But the body can store only so much glycogen. When the storehouses are full, the excess is converted to fat for storage. While glycogen can be converted back to glucose for quick energy when blood glucose levels become too low, fat cannot be changed back to glucose.

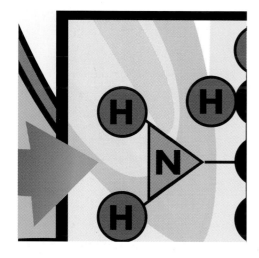

CHAPTER 2

Protein: Brain, Growth, Healing . . . and Living Power

LEGEND HAS IT that every day sixth-century Greek Olympic wrestler Miles of Crotona ate 20 pounds of meat and lifted a growing calf, essentially practicing progressive resistance training. When the calf reached four years of age, Miles carried it the length of Olympia stadium, killed, roasted, and ate it.

Although we now know that eating extra protein doesn't make extra muscle, to the disappointment of many athletes, we also know that protein is critical to life. At work in every cell of the body, protein is the most important nutrient supporting growth and tissue repair. It also drives the body's never-ending chemical reactions that make us breathe, keep our heart beating, and stimulate every other action vital to life. Without protein, our hormones, antibodies (essential to fighting infections), and genes (the body's code for making any tissue or cell) could not function. Proteins play at least two other roles: They are essential in keeping the chemical mix of the blood optimal for good health, and if the body experiences an energy crisis—if it doesn't take in enough calories—it can burn protein as energy, albeit less efficiently and with more unwanted by-products than when it burns carbohydrates.

It's no wonder that protein derives its name from the Greek *proteios,* meaning "holding first place."

Protein is constructed of building blocks called amino acids. Like carbohydrates and fats (as you'll read in Chapter 3), amino acids are made of carbon, hydrogen, and oxygen molecules. But an additional element, nitrogen, distinguishes protein from these other energy sources.

All amino acids are joined together in thousands of ways to form long chains called peptides. Two proteins may have totally different functions—liver protein and muscle protein, for example—but be composed of exactly the same amino acids. The difference lies in how these amino acids are linked together.

There are two categories of amino acids: essential and nonessential. These categories have nothing to do with how important each is in the human body. Rather, the categories distinguish those amino acids the body can make from those it cannot. Of the 22 amino acids needed by the human body, 9 are dietary *essentials*, or must be gotten through the diet; the remaining 13 are *nonessential* dietary components because the body can make them from scraps of left-over carbohydrates, fats, and other amino acids.

If you lack just one essential amino acid for any period of time—no matter what quantity of other amino acids you eat—your body will break down your own muscle tissue to harvest that essential amino acid it needs to build hormones and perform functions less vital than building and maintaining muscle tissue. If this process continues, you may suffer the effects of protein malnutrition, which, in addition to loss of muscle mass, include thin, fragile hair (or hair loss); skin sores; swelling; and one or many chemical and hormonal imbalances. Fortunately, protein deficiency of this severity is rare in the United States.

Body proteins are in a constant state of flux. Not only is the protein we eat broken down to its constituent amino acids, but body proteins are constantly being disassembled and reassembled. Muscle proteins, for example, are broken down and quickly re-formed into muscle tissue as well as into other protein-containing tissues and cells. In this process, called protein turnover, most of the amino acids are re-formed into other (nonessential) amino acids and then assimilated into body proteins. Some, however, are discarded. That's why dietary protein, which replaces these discarded amino acids, is just as important in old age as it is to rapidly growing babies.

Protein-containing foods can be divided into two main categories, complete proteins and incomplete proteins, based on what kinds of amino acids they contain, or their amino acid mix. Foods containing all essential amino acids are called complete proteins. If one or more essential amino acids are lacking, that protein is termed incomplete. While most protein from animal sources—milk, cheese, eggs, meat, fish, and poultry—is complete, most protein from plant sources is incomplete. Other foods, such as soybeans and many nuts, can be said to be "weakly complete"; that is, they contain all essential amino acids, but they don't have enough of one or more essential amino acids to assemble body proteins. Fortunately, though, these incomplete or weakly complete protein foods can be used as complete protein sources.

With a little dietary maneuvering, one incomplete protein food can be combined with another incomplete protein food chosen to make up for the other's deficiency. This is called *complementing* proteins. The trick is to make correct combinations. Until recently, nutrition experts thought incomplete proteins had to be complemented within the same meal to ensure their use as protein rather than fuel. More recent research, however, reveals that incomplete protein foods only need to be complemented within a day's time. The following pages show how incomplete protein foods can be combined to supply high-quality, complete protein. Eating a very small quantity of a complete protein food with an incomplete one—a glass of milk with a peanut butter sandwich, for example—also ensures that the protein in the incomplete protein food will be converted to a high-quality protein.

As important as protein is to the body, it is often misunderstood. Misconceptions include those leading us to consume too much protein, too little protein, avoid protein from certain sources altogether, or pop amino acid pills.

The story of Miles of Crotona illustrates well the myth that extra protein is the ticket to building extra muscle tissue. Unfortunately, extra protein doesn't form extra muscle, and worse yet, it cannot be stored for later use. Instead, it is burned as fuel or metabolized and stored as fat. Dealing with this extra protein is not as easy as it sounds. Not only is this practice expensive (adding extra meat, cheese, and fish to your diet quickly raises your grocery bill), but it can strain the body's metabolic machinery.

Consider this analogy. While burning natural gas is a great source of energy with few by-products, burning your grandmother's mahogany dining room table to heat the house isn't such a great idea. While it would produce heat, this heat is produced at great cost and also, because of the stain and finish, generates nasty by-products. The unwanted by-products of burning protein for energy must pass through the kidneys to be excreted through the urine. While most people can handle these by-products, others cannot. In addition, if you eat excess protein in the form of meat, you may be getting far more fat and cholesterol than you bargained for. And here's one other negative consequence of eating too much animal protein: Such a diet causes the body to lose excessive amounts of the mineral calcium that is so critical to building strong bones and teeth.

While body builders frequently eat too much protein, other athletes, especially women endurance athletes, shun protein to load up on carbohydrates. Having heard that carbohydrates will improve their performance, they've fashioned diets of pasta, salad, bagels, and, well, more pasta. Like Miles, they are carrying a good thing too far. Sports nutrition experts say some such women are actually protein deficient, as evidenced by a gray cast to their skin, brittle hair, brittle nails, and amenorrhea, or the cessation of the menstrual period. One study found that 82% of amenorrheic athletes ate less than the recommended dietary allowance of protein.

There's another critical point about protein: You have to eat enough calories in order to use dietary protein *as* protein—this is called "sparing" protein. If you're terribly short on calories, you'll simply burn protein for energy (this is one reason not to crash diet—see Chapter 16).

More and more people shun eggs and red meat. Because of their high cholesterol and/or fat content, they stand falsely accused of being bad foods. A healthier approach is to blend small amounts of these foods into your weekly diet, alternating them with other protein sources. Getting your protein through a variety of foods also ensures that you'll get other essential nutrients. Red meat, for example, is high in iron and zinc, which are difficult to get through other foods. Dairy foods are high in calcium.

One of the more dangerous protein myths concerns amino acid supplements, which are sold without a prescription in drug and health food stores. Over the years, various amino acids have been touted as cure-alls for many ailments. Methionine is sold to improve the liver's ability to neutralize toxins; lysine was once promoted as a herpes cure. Neither claim has ever been proven. Nor is there any truth to the belief that amino acid supplements help athletes build muscle and perform better. While they are most likely just expensive calorie sources, amino acid supplements may be harmful, especially in large doses. Excessive amounts may cause diarrhea and dehydration, and there is some evidence that they may cause an amino acid imbalance. In 1974, the Food and Drug Administration removed amino acid supplements from their list of substances "generally recognized as safe" (the GRAS list).

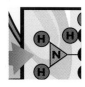

How much protein do you need? Much less than many people in America eat. Many Americans consume twice the amount they need to be healthy. Most people need to eat just 8% to 10% of their daily calories as protein (although dietary guidelines are set at 10% to 15% to be on the safe side). Growing children, pregnant women, and nursing mothers need a little more, as do people recovering from a serious illness or injury.

What does this mean in real food terms? The average adult can get enough protein for a day with 3 ounces of meat (half a chicken breast), a slice of bread, 1 cup of milk, and 2 ounces of cheese; vegetarians can substitute 2 cups of legumes (lentils, kidney beans, or pinto beans).

Mathematically speaking, every day you need 0.8 grams of protein for every kilogram of body weight (1 kilogram is equal to 2.2 pounds). Using the example of a 170-pound man, here's how you can calculate your own protein requirement:

170 pounds ÷ 2.2 = 77.3 kilograms

77.3 kilograms × 0.8 = 62 grams protein

62 grams protein × 4 calories/gram = 248 calories of protein

Remember that you can't just weigh a protein food to determine the number of grams of protein it has. Packaged into foods high in protein are many other things that account for part of the weight, including water, fat, and in plant sources of protein, carbohydrates. On average, an ounce of meat, fish, poultry, or cheese has 7 grams of protein, and ½ cup of cooked lentils and other dried beans and peas has 8 grams.

If you've been planning your meals around a meat (or fish or poultry) main course, consider using these high-protein sources as a side dish. Instead, feature complex carbohydrates (as outlined in Chapter 1), fruits, and vegetables as the main part of your meal. Three ounces of meat is just the size of a deck of playing cards, which looks awfully small when there are few other items on your plate. This new way of thinking about meat will help you reap the benefits of good nutrition and great health.

How Nature Makes Protein

Breaking apart the building blocks of protein, amino acids, reveals a fascinating fact: They are formed from carbon, hydrogen, and oxygen, the same basic elements that form carbohydrates and fat. But nature distinguishes protein by adding nitrogen, another naturally occurring element. Many amino acids contain other elements, including sulfur, phosphorus, iron, and iodine. Read on to see how all animals depend on plants and microorganisms to form protein building blocks.

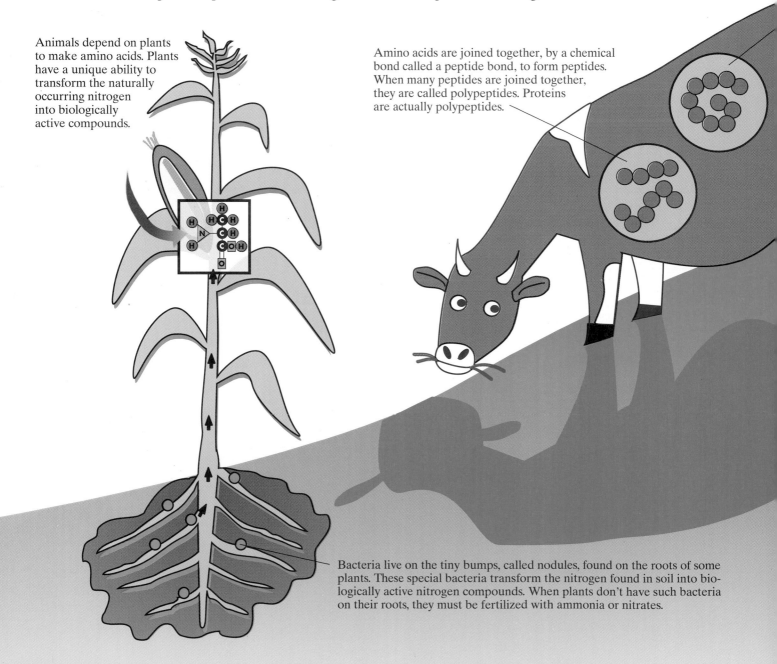

Animals depend on plants to make amino acids. Plants have a unique ability to transform the naturally occurring nitrogen into biologically active compounds.

Amino acids are joined together, by a chemical bond called a peptide bond, to form peptides. When many peptides are joined together, they are called polypeptides. Proteins are actually polypeptides.

Bacteria live on the tiny bumps, called nodules, found on the roots of some plants. These special bacteria transform the nitrogen found in soil into biologically active nitrogen compounds. When plants don't have such bacteria on their roots, they must be fertilized with ammonia or nitrates.

When animals eat plants, they disassemble the protein contained in the plants into its constituent amino acids via digestion. They can then make whatever amino acids they need to live by reformulating the amino acids into other polypeptides.

People must get all essential amino acids from either animal protein or the correct combination of plant foods. Nonessential amino acids can be made by reformulating amino acids from any protein source, as well as from leftover scraps of carbohydrate, protein, and fat.

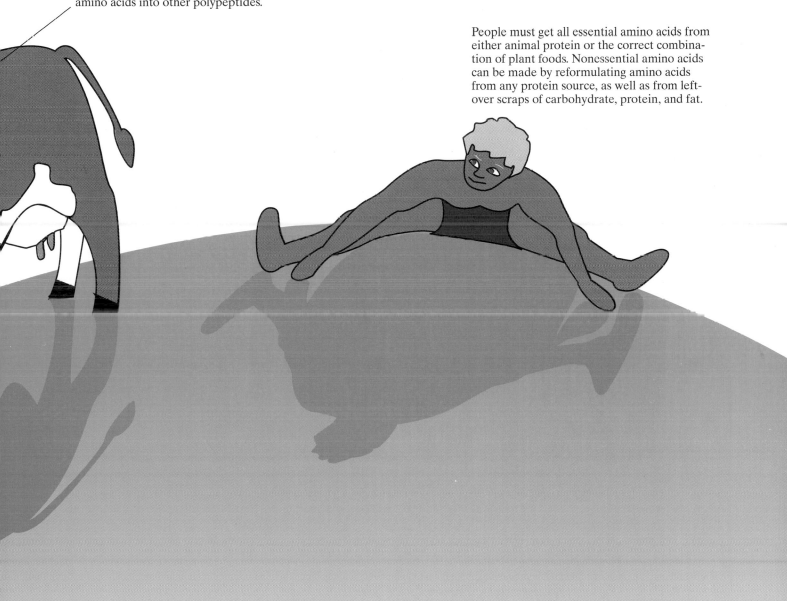

How the Body Uses Protein

Protein is essential every minute of our lives—from the moment of conception to our last day. In its many and varied forms, protein makes our heart beat, powers our brain cells, makes our muscles contract to keep us moving, fights infections, heals cuts, and performs or drives countless other tasks.

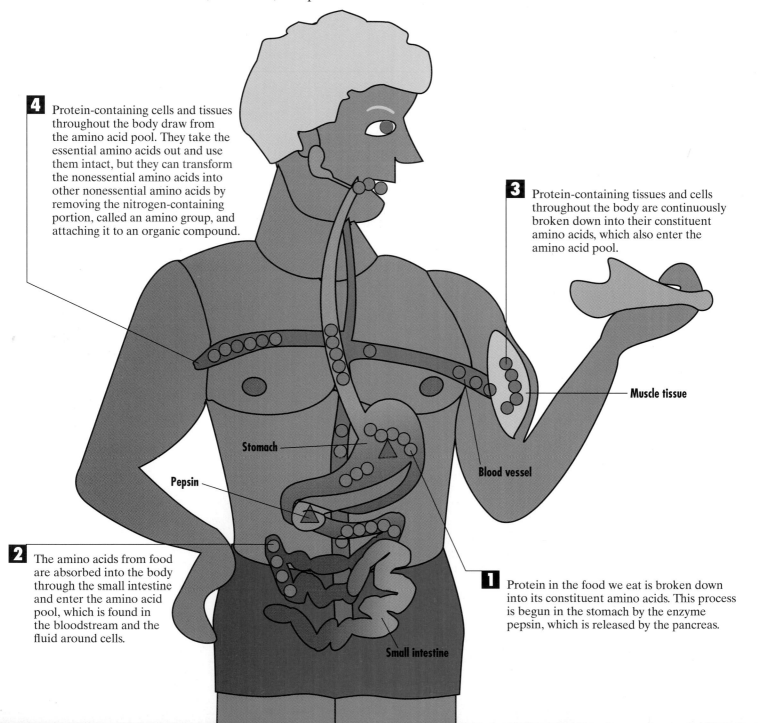

4 Protein-containing cells and tissues throughout the body draw from the amino acid pool. They take the essential amino acids out and use them intact, but they can transform the nonessential amino acids into other nonessential amino acids by removing the nitrogen-containing portion, called an amino group, and attaching it to an organic compound.

3 Protein-containing tissues and cells throughout the body are continuously broken down into their constituent amino acids, which also enter the amino acid pool.

Muscle tissue

Stomach

Pepsin

Blood vessel

2 The amino acids from food are absorbed into the body through the small intestine and enter the amino acid pool, which is found in the bloodstream and the fluid around cells.

1 Protein in the food we eat is broken down into its constituent amino acids. This process is begun in the stomach by the enzyme pepsin, which is released by the pancreas.

Small intestine

Proteins are found in every cell throughout the body. Here we note just a small fraction of the many thousands necessary to keep us alive and well.

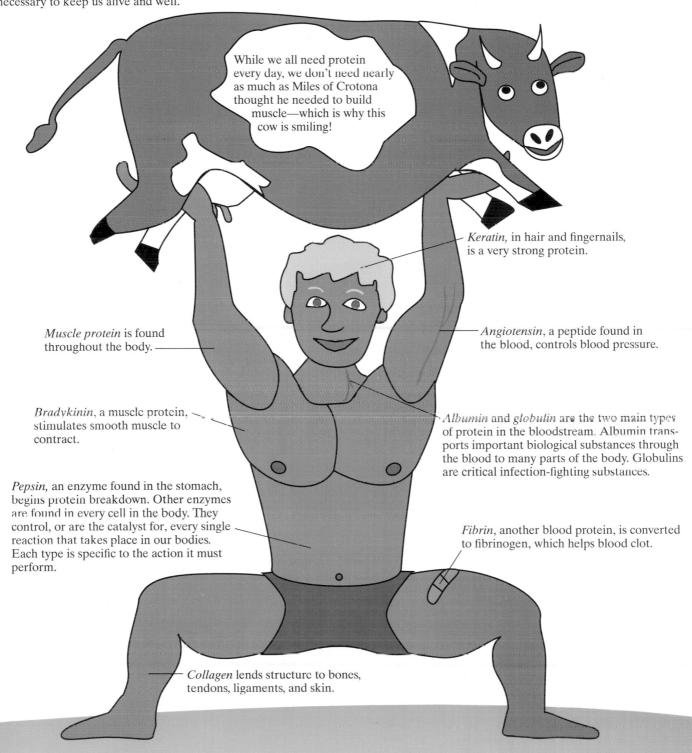

While we all need protein every day, we don't need nearly as much as Miles of Crotona thought he needed to build muscle—which is why this cow is smiling!

Keratin, in hair and fingernails, is a very strong protein.

Muscle protein is found throughout the body.

Angiotensin, a peptide found in the blood, controls blood pressure.

Bradykinin, a muscle protein, stimulates smooth muscle to contract.

Albumin and *globulin* are the two main types of protein in the bloodstream. Albumin transports important biological substances through the blood to many parts of the body. Globulins are critical infection-fighting substances.

Pepsin, an enzyme found in the stomach, begins protein breakdown. Other enzymes are found in every cell in the body. They control, or are the catalyst for, every single reaction that takes place in our bodies. Each type is specific to the action it must perform.

Fibrin, another blood protein, is converted to fibrinogen, which helps blood clot.

Collagen lends structure to bones, tendons, ligaments, and skin.

Many Combinations Can Make a Day's Worth of Complete Protein

If you're like most Americans, you tend to think just of meat, poultry, and fish as good protein sources. As you see by the choices here, you're in for another adventure in eating when you mix up your diet with some of these other great protein foods. Variety in food choices brings you one step closer to harvesting all the nutrients you need for great health!

Animal Sources   These foods supply the highest-quality protein, or complete protein foods containing all essential amino acids. There are three subclasses of animal protein: milk and milk products; eggs; and meat, poultry, and fish. In addition to protein, each supplies a different mix of other nutrients. Dairy products also provide B-12 and phosphorus. Pork and beef are prime sources of iron and zinc, and great sources of phosphorus and many B vitamins. Fish has a naturally occurring oil that may help fight heart disease.

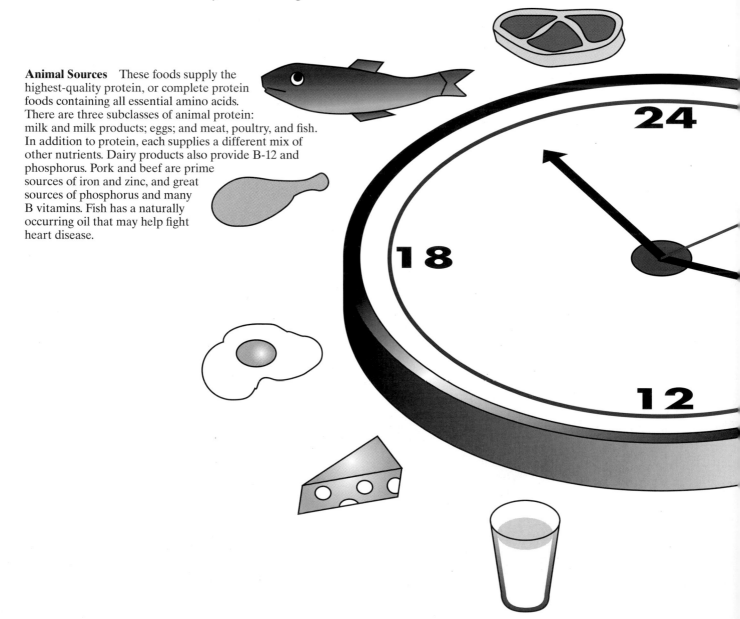

Plant sources   With the rare exception, plant foods don't contain all essential amino acids, making them incomplete protein foods. Combine plant foods as suggested below to make complete proteins. These foods are also loaded with complex carbohydrates, fiber, and a different mix of vitamins and minerals than found in meat sources of protein.

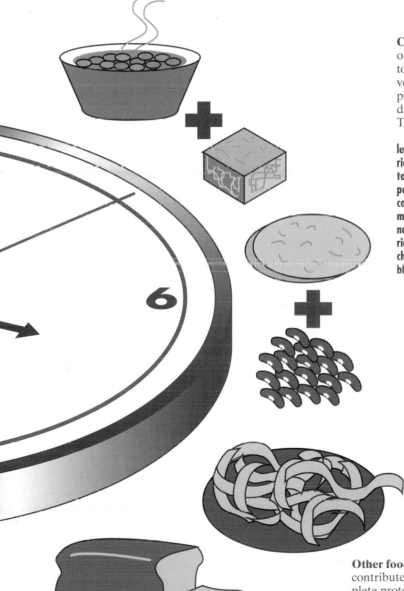

Complementing proteins   The incomplete protein in one plant food can be combined with that of another to yield a complete protein, in a little dietary maneuvering called complementing proteins. Incomplete protein foods only need to be complemented within a day's time, not at each meal as was previously thought. The following combinations make complete proteins.

lentil soup + corn bread
rice + kidney beans
tofu + rice
peanut butter + whole wheat bread
corn tortilla + pinto beans
meatless chili + whole wheat bread
navy beans + rye bread
rice cakes + peanut butter
chick peas + corn bread
black-eyed peas + corn bread

Other foods   Pasta, breads, and bagels also contribute some protein to the diet. The complete proteins you consume in a day's time ensure that the incomplete proteins these foods contain will be used as protein when needed.

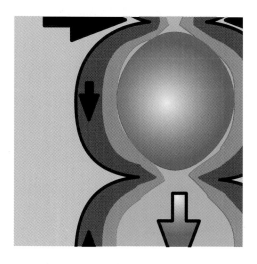

CHAPTER
3

Fat: Both Friend and Foe

WITHOUT IT, THE body's millions upon billions of cells could neither form properly nor regulate the entry and exit of nutrients, hormones, and other life-essential chemicals. Vital internal organs might suffer serious injury in its absence. Hormones couldn't form or function, nor could the body harness, transport, and use certain vitamins without it.

The mystery substance? Fat—a term we've come to despise and a substance we try to avoid as though it were the plague. But fat performs all the vital functions just described. It also lends intense flavor and mouth-pleasing texture to food and keeps us feeling full and satisfied for hours longer than its energy-supplying cohorts, protein and carbohydrates. Fat is also the most compact source of energy.

Unfortunately, fat is as overconsumed as it is necessary to life and good health. In fact, eating too much fat is the single most important dietary mistake made in this country. As a nation, we eat some 839 billion fat calories each year. But in the fervor to reduce dietary fat, Americans are forgetting a crucial fact: It's the dose that makes the poison. Consider this analogy: Aspirin can lower a fever and relieve pain at the right dose, but it's harmful at higher doses. The same is true of many nutrients and chemicals. Too much salt and even too much water can be fatal. But they, like fat, are crucial to the human body.

Chemically speaking, fat is just one substance within a larger category of substances called lipids. Oily or greasy to the touch and insoluble in water, lipids include dietary fats such as cooking oil, butter, lard, and the fat that is an inherent part of many meats, dairy products, and other foods. Also included under the lipid umbrella are hormones, waxes, and sterols. Cholesterol is the best-known sterol. Not a dietary fat at all, it's a fatlike substance present in all animal cells. Cholesterol does not supply calories because it is not composed of the same energy-supplying compounds that fats and oils are. Surprisingly, the majority of the cholesterol in our bodies is formed within the body itself from substances other than dietary cholesterol.

Fat is formed from the same basic ingredients found in nature as are protein and carbohydrates: carbon, hydrogen, and oxygen. The difference is in the proportions and how they're connected. Fats contain much less oxygen than do proteins and carbohydrates. Simply put, the air is squeezed out of fat, which makes it a more compact source of energy. That is because fats provide 9 calories per gram, over twice as many as each gram of protein and carbohydrate.

Dietary fats consist mainly of triglycerides, which are made up of one glycerol molecule connected to three fatty acids. The most important structural feature of a triglyceride is the fatty acid portion. This is the segment that distinguishes one type of triglyceride, or dietary fat, from the other, both in terms of flavor and the fat's effect within the human body. Some fatty acids are saturated, some are monounsaturated, and others are polyunsaturated. Saturation simply has to do with how much hydrogen a fat contains. Saturated fatty acids are saturated with hydrogen, or contain the maximum amount of hydrogen possible. Fats missing one pair of hydrogen atoms are monounsaturated; those missing more than one pair are polyunsaturated. Although they differ by just a couple of hydrogen atoms, these different types of fat behave quite differently in the body (see Chapter 13).

The body can make most fatty acids from carbon, hydrogen, and oxygen atoms left over from any excess fat, protein, or carbohydrate foods consumed. But three fatty acids cannot be made in the body and are therefore called essential fatty acids. The body needs essential fatty acids to construct healthy cell walls, make cholesterol (believe it or not, the body needs cholesterol to function normally, as you'll see on the following page), and to make substances called prostaglandins that regulate blood pressure, blood clotting, and other functions critical to life. The essential fatty acids are linoleic, arachidonic, and linolenic. If your diet contains enough linoleic acid, the body can make the other two essential fatty acids from it.

How much fat do we need to be healthy? As is true with protein, much less than many people consume! Just 20 grams of dietary fat a day meets the body's requirement. More specifically, we need to consume just polyunsaturated fat, which is where essential fatty acids are found. If you think about it, this must be one way nature tries to protect us. It is saturated fat, which is unessential to the body, that wreaks the most havoc on our health.

Many Americans consume closer to 100 grams of dietary fat per day, and much of that, unfortunately, is in the form of saturated fat. Put another way, the average American consumes nearly 4 of every 10 calories as fat, when 3 of every 10 is the maximum recommended. Lowering this to around 2 of every 10 calories (which is still more than we actually need) confers even greater health benefits, especially when that fat is primarily in the form of polyunsaturated and monounsaturated fatty acids.

Why do we get into so much trouble with dietary fat? Some of the strengths of dietary fat quickly become its weaknesses. That full-bodied flavor makes it difficult to limit foods containing fat. Their caloric density, an advantage during an energy crisis, also gets us into trouble quickly; just a little taste generally delivers a lot of calories. In addition, some of the easiest foods to grab in a hurry—fast foods and convenience foods—are often laced with lots of fat, especially saturated fat. And some fast foods as well as many other foods contain fat that we can't readily see or taste, which makes it even more difficult to avoid.

Eating too much fat gets you into many health troubles. Gaining too much weight is prime among them. Unfortunately, a calorie is not a calorie as far as the body's energy-storing apparatus is concerned. As we mentioned in Chapter 1, excess fat calories are stored with much greater ease and at a much lower energy cost than are excess carbo-hydrate calories. Where the body burns up 25 of every 100 extra carbohydrate calories in the process of trying to store those calories for later use, just 3 calories of energy are needed to pack away 100 extra fat calories. Put another way, fat calories are more fat-tening than carbohydrate calories. Being overweight puts you at risk of many health problems, including high blood pressure (and consequently stroke), high blood choles-terol, adult-onset diabetes, and arthritis and other joint problems. Eating too much dietary fat may also contribute to the development of cancer, heart disease, and stroke.

No doubt you've heard about trans fatty acids, and you're wondering if you've been sold a bill of goods about margarine all these years: Is butter actually more healthful than margarine? But what are these trans fatty acids anyway? Remember that significant structural feature of triglycerides, the fatty acid portion—the portion that distinguishes one type of fat from another? In the process of making margarine from oil, those fatty acids are transformed. More specifically, polyunsaturated oils are rendered into solids by adding some of the missing hydrogen atoms back into the polyunsaturated structure in a process call hydrogenation. If you were to look at the fatty acid in three dimensions before and after hydrogenation, you would see that the hydrogenation process changes the fatty acid configuration from its original *cis* form (in scientist's lingo) to a *trans* form, the form that has come under fire. Although the final verdict isn't in, research suggests that trans fatty acids behave somewhat like saturated fatty acids—which means they may play some role in increasing the levels of LDL (bad)-cholesterol. But let's put this news into perspective: If you follow the dietary guidelines suggested in this book, and limit the amount of fat you eat, a little trans (or even saturated) fat isn't "bad" for you. It's the quantity—or as we said earlier in this chapter, it's the dose that makes the poison. The best advice is to cut fat intake overall, choosing liquid forms of monounsaturated cooking oils (peanut, canola, olive) whenever a recipe does call for cooking fat. Try alternative toppings for your bagels, potatoes, and vegetables, such as jams, nonfat sour cream, and lemon juice.

On the next pages, we'll go to the market with the policeman on fat detail, who will show us sections of the grocery store that are relatively low in fat, versus those that are full of fat land mines and in which you have to choose carefully.

Sources of Fat: Stop, Go, Proceed with Caution

Just 40% to 50% of the fat we eat is visible to the naked eye. Examples are the fat we see circling a cut of meat or marbled within; the margarine, butter, or cream cheese we spread on toast and bagels; and the salad dressing we slather on our greens. The rest is invisible, or hidden. Here, the policeman on fat duty accompanies us through the grocery store, pointing out potential fat land mines. In green-light areas, choose foods freely; in yellow, you'll have to read labels and choose carefully. The majority of foods in red-light areas quickly break anyone's fat budget.

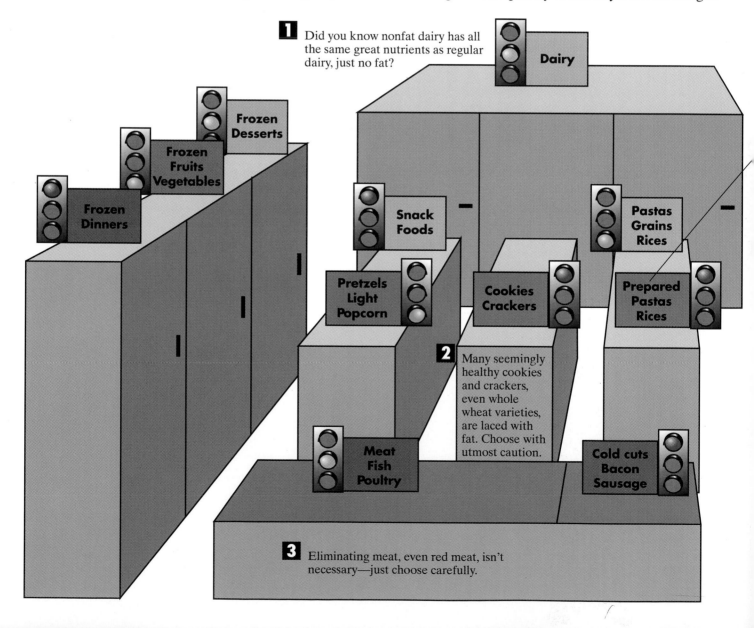

1 Did you know nonfat dairy has all the same great nutrients as regular dairy, just no fat?

Dairy

Frozen Desserts

Frozen Fruits Vegetables

Frozen Dinners

Snack Foods

Pastas Grains Rices

Pretzels Light Popcorn

Cookies Crackers

Prepared Pastas Rices

2 Many seemingly healthy cookies and crackers, even whole wheat varieties, are laced with fat. Choose with utmost caution.

Meat Fish Poultry

Cold cuts Bacon Sausage

3 Eliminating meat, even red meat, isn't necessary—just choose carefully.

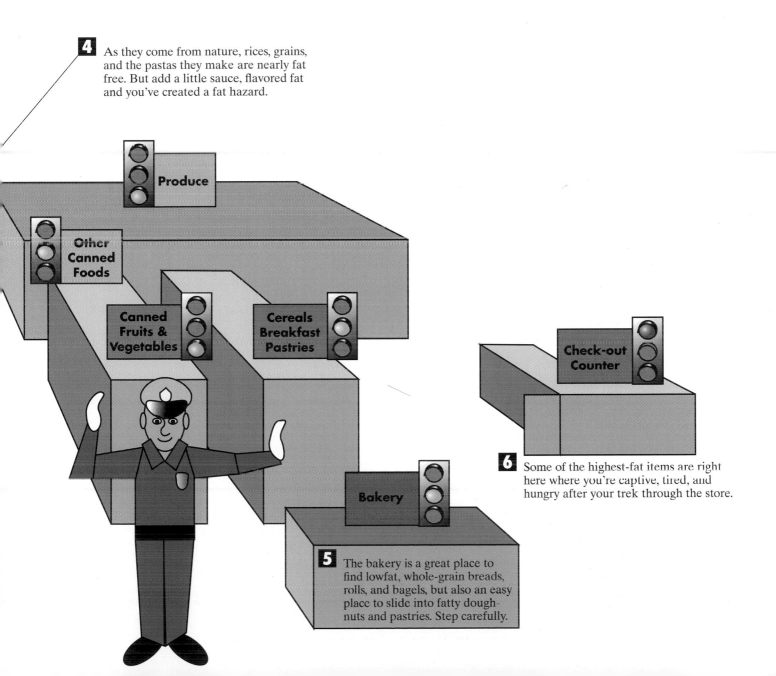

4 As they come from nature, rices, grains, and the pastas they make are nearly fat free. But add a little sauce, flavored fat and you've created a fat hazard.

Produce

Other Canned Foods

Canned Fruits & Vegetables

Cereals Breakfast Pastries

Check-out Counter

6 Some of the highest-fat items are right here where you're captive, tired, and hungry after your trek through the store.

Bakery

5 The bakery is a great place to find lowfat, whole-grain breads, rolls, and bagels, but also an easy place to slide into fatty dough-nuts and pastries. Step carefully.

How the Body Uses Fat

Although fat has been villainized, we couldn't live without it. Dietary fat is converted to many types of lipids, which are found in every cell in the body and are the basis for many vital regulatory processes. Here we distinguish those functions for which dietary fat is essential, seen on the left side of the page, from those on the right, which require fat that can be formed within the body from any carbon, oxygen, and hydrogen atoms—from left-over proteins and carbohydrates, for example.

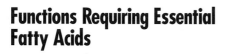

Functions Requiring Essential Fatty Acids

Absorbs Vitamin A Ingredient   Carrots and certain other nonfat vegetables contain a chemical called beta-carotene, which is converted to vitamin A inside the body. We cannot absorb these vitamin A precursors, as they are called, without dietary fat. In general, dietary fat is essential for the absorption of all fat-soluble vitamins, A, D, E, and K. In this picture, the fingerlike projections are microscopic cells inside the intestine responsible for absorbing food.

Transports Vitamins   Without fat, the fat-soluble vitamins could not be carried in the bloodstream to where they are needed in the body. Eating just 20 grams of fat per day meets this requirement.

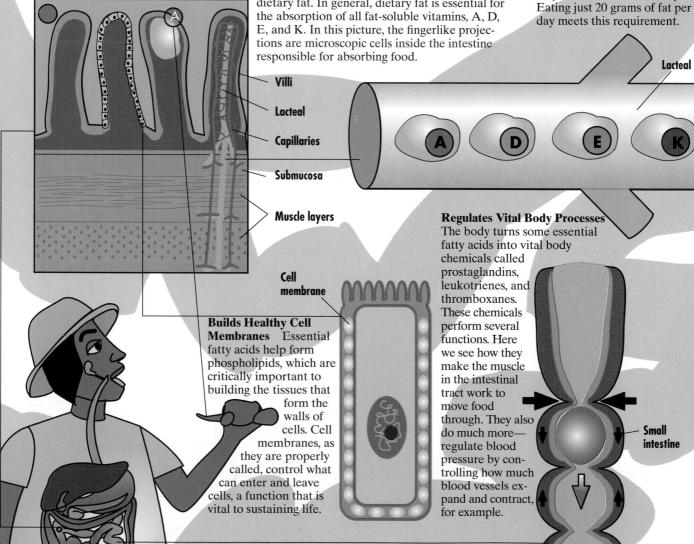

Villi

Lacteal

Capillaries

Submucosa

Muscle layers

Lacteal

A D E K

Cell membrane

Builds Healthy Cell Membranes   Essential fatty acids help form phospholipids, which are critically important to building the tissues that form the walls of cells. Cell membranes, as they are properly called, control what can enter and leave cells, a function that is vital to sustaining life.

Regulates Vital Body Processes
The body turns some essential fatty acids into vital body chemicals called prostaglandins, leukotrienes, and thromboxanes. These chemicals perform several functions. Here we see how they make the muscle in the intestinal tract work to move food through. They also do much more—regulate blood pressure by controlling how much blood vessels expand and contract, for example.

Small intestine

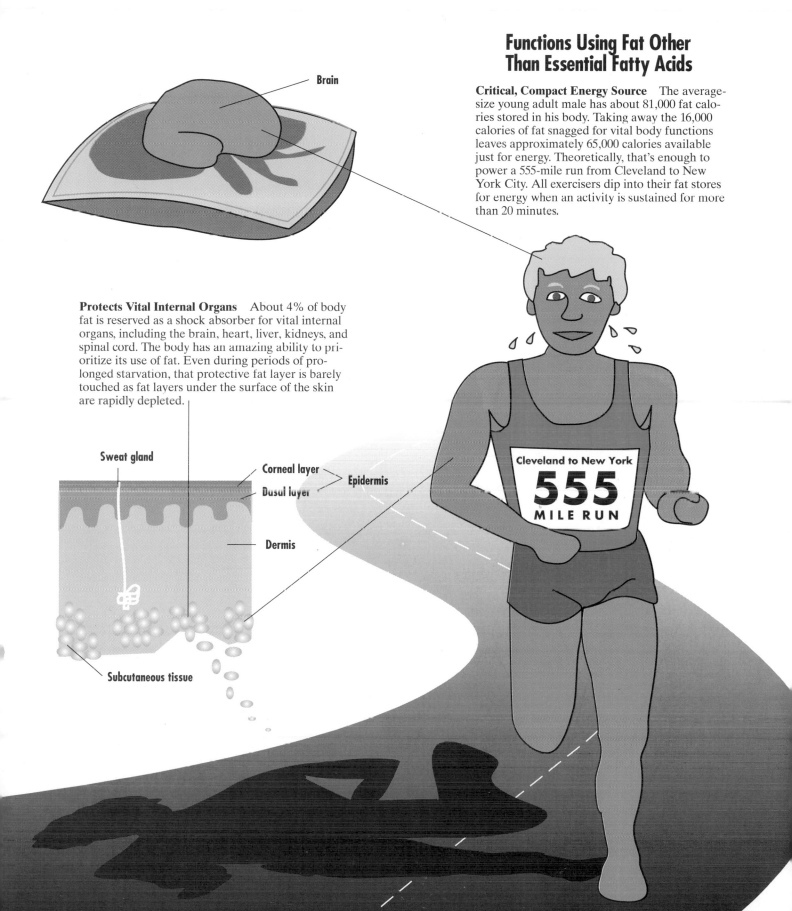

Brain

Functions Using Fat Other Than Essential Fatty Acids

Critical, Compact Energy Source The average-size young adult male has about 81,000 fat calories stored in his body. Taking away the 16,000 calories of fat snagged for vital body functions leaves approximately 65,000 calories available just for energy. Theoretically, that's enough to power a 555-mile run from Cleveland to New York City. All exercisers dip into their fat stores for energy when an activity is sustained for more than 20 minutes.

Protects Vital Internal Organs About 4% of body fat is reserved as a shock absorber for vital internal organs, including the brain, heart, liver, kidneys, and spinal cord. The body has an amazing ability to prioritize its use of fat. Even during periods of prolonged starvation, that protective fat layer is barely touched as fat layers under the surface of the skin are rapidly depleted.

Sweat gland

Corneal layer

Dusul layer

Epidermis

Dermis

Subcutaneous tissue

Cleveland to New York

555
MILE RUN

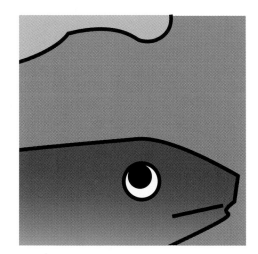

Balancing Macronutrients for Awesome Health

A CALORIE IS A calorie is a calorie? Not exactly. By now you've learned that the three macro- or calorie-supplying nutrients, carbohydrate, protein, and fat, weren't created equal—especially in what they contribute to your body's growth, energy, and metabolic needs. It's not enough to count calories, just trying to stay within a reasonable limit to achieve or maintain a trim weight. You owe it your health to think about where calories come from, making sure you get the optimal fuel mix to power, grow, and repair every cell in your body. Protein calories are no substitute for carbohydrate calories, which are no substitute for fat calories. Would you think of refueling your car with kerosene? Definitely not! Begin to think of your body as a machine that is just as fussy as your car or lawn mower about what kind of fuel it gets.

What's the best fuel mix? Health and nutrition experts recommend we limit fat calories to no more than 30% of a day's total calories, reserve 10%–15% for protein, and aim for 55%–60% in carbohydrates. But you're not alone if you have no idea how to translate this bit of information into shopping carts of food and then onto plates at mealtime.

First of all, it's only the rare food that is purely one type of macronutrient or another. Sugar, honey, and corn syrup, for example, are pure carbohydrate calories, and margarine, butter, and oils are pure fat calories. But most foods have varying combinations of macronutrients.

Most protein calories are woven into a bundle containing fat and carbohydrate, the proportions varying by food source. Vegetable sources of protein, such as lentils and navy beans, are high in carbohydrate and low in fat, while animal sources of protein are high in fat and have almost no carbohydrate (except milk and other dairy foods). Most complex-carbohydrate foods are naturally free of fat, while many simple carbohydrate treats (such as candy bars) are made with lots of extra fat. In other words, you can't just choose a diet of 3 parts fat foods, 1–1½ parts protein foods, and 5½–6parts carbohydrate foods.

Short of taking a calculator and some food guides to the grocery store, how does the average person figure out what to eat to achieve this optimal fuel mix?

While the following advice may seem revolutionary, it's actually as old as humankind. Throw away the calculator and the food guides. Instead, think of food in categories, and choose it in forms as close as possible to the the way you'd find it in nature. Put another way, think about filling your grocery cart from foods that commonly line the edges of the grocery store—the produce, dairy, bakery, meat, fish, and poultry sections—and the aisles containing cereal, cereal grains, legumes, rices, pastas, flours and nuts.

Linger long in the produce aisle, browsing through and choosing nature's most beautifully painted foods for each meal of the day: Choose a different fruit for each meal, and select at least one vegetable for lunch and dinner, aiming for different choices each day of the week. Then toss in enough interesting fruit for between-meal snacks. If the produce selections are wanting, turn to the frozen food or canned food aisle, choosing items without added fat, sauce, or salt.

In the dairy section, opt for low- or nonfat milk, yogurt, sour cream, and cream cheese. Choose lower-fat cheeses, or those with 3–5 grams of fat per ounce, keeping in mind that nonfat cheeses don't always have acceptable taste or texture. Don't shy away from eggs if you like them; they're an excellent lowfat source of protein.

In the bakery, gather whole- or coarse-grain breads and bagels, and add in whole-grain, fruited muffins for an occasional treat.

At the meat, fish, and poultry case, buy no more than 4–6 ounces (uncooked) per person per day. A family of four, for example, can have a dinner of hamburgers from a pound of raw hamburger. Choose some of each type of flesh foods—pork, beef, fish, and poultry—each week. See the following pages on how to choose lower-fat versions and how to balance these foods.

For breakfast foods, choose whole-grain cereals such as oatmeal or a cereal high in fiber.

For lunches, gather an interesting combination of legumes, lentils, and nuts; you can turn them into split-pea soup, lentil-nut salad, or meatless chili. Choose enough so that you'll have a vegetable source of protein for two nights of the week.

Choose "a grain a day," or a different grain for each night of the week. Purchase enough so that you're eating more grains and other starches than flesh food at any given meal. For example, alternate brown rice, couscous, millet, quinoa, whole-wheat berries, bulgur, barley, potatoes, and pastas, or combine them to make interesting pilafs and casseroles.

For cooking oil, choose olive, peanut, or canola oil, and for accents turn to interesting spices, vinegars, lowfat salad dressings, mustards, relishes, fresh herbs, broths, gourmet marmalades, and dried fruits.

If you fill your grocery cart using these guidelines, you'll have gathered foods that will meet the recommendation of getting 30% of your calories from fat, 10%–15% from protein, and 55%–60% from carbohydrate. And you'll be pleasantly surprised when the cashier rings up a smaller total grocery bill!

As you think about organizing your food for the week, remember this additional critical advice: At lunch and dinner, fill two-thirds of your plate with complex carbohydrates, which means including 1–3 servings of grains, breads, pastas and/or potatoes (depending on your age and size), 1–2 vegetable servings, and 1 fruit serving at each meal (where a serving is ½ cup—the amount that fits into the palm of your hand—or one whole fruit or vegetable). Put another way, if you're the typical American, double up on grains, fruits, and vegetables.

Limit your meat (including cheese and eggs in this total) portion to 3–5 ounces (cooked) per day. A 3-ounce serving is about the size of a deck of playing cards or the palm (not including the fingers) of a woman's hand. As a general rule, choose 3 ounces of meat (or fish or poultry) at dinner, and a vegetable source of protein at lunch. Again, if you're the typical American, halve your protein serving to achieve a healthier-sized portion.

Also remember to do the following: Cook food in as little monounsaturated oil as possible, steaming vegetables and sautéing in a mixture of oil and broth; daily add in 2–4 servings of nonfat or lowfat dairy foods, such as milk and yogurt; and snack from your produce bins, fruit bowl, and whole-grain breadbasket. With this simple advice, you'll get the fuel mix you need from your grocery cart.

One other piece of advice to make this work: Balancing your appetite is just as important as balancing your nutrients. Plan in one generous serving of a special, gooey dessert one night each week. Cheesecake, key lime pie, or hot fudge sundae—whatever strikes your fancy, plan to have it each week. That's how the real world eats and still maintains an awesome nutrition profile—and trim waistline.

Dividing Your Daily Calories among the Macronutrients

The body craves just the right mix of fuel to perform maximally: about 12% to 15% as protein, no more than 30% as fat, and about 55% to 60% as carbohydrate. Use the Reference Diet to convert those numbers into real food groups, based on your age and sex.

The Reference Diet

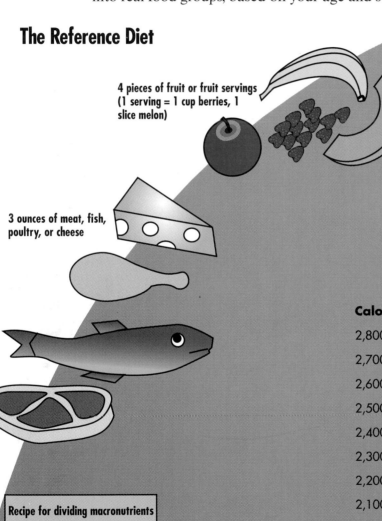

4 pieces of fruit or fruit servings (1 serving = 1 cup berries, 1 slice melon)

6 bread or starch servings (1 serving =1 slice bread, ½ bagel, ½ cup rice or pasta, ½ baked potato)

3 ounces of meat, fish, poultry, or cheese

Young women aged 15–22 need around 2,100 calories. To add calories to the reference diet in the right proportions, they should add the foods listed below. Young men aged 15–22 have incredible energy needs, some 2,800 calories each day. But they also need to balance their macronutrients. They should add the foods listed below.

Recipe for dividing macronutrients

1½ parts protein

3 parts fat

5½ parts carbohydrates

Calories Needed

	Female	Male
2,800		
2,700		
2,600		
2,500		
2,400		
2,300		Reference Diet plus:
2,200		2 oz. meat or fish or...
2,100	Reference Diet plus:	4 bread/starch
2,000	1 oz. meat or fish or...	2 low-fat milk
1,900	2 bread/starch	2 fat
1,800	1 low-fat milk	1 c. legumes

15–22 years old

The Reference Diet (illustrated here) is designed for the population group with the lowest calorie needs—women over the age of 50. Depending on your age and sex, add to this Reference Diet to bring you calories up to the level you need—in just the right proportions. If you want to lose weight, refer to Chapter 16 for how to adjust the Reference Diet.

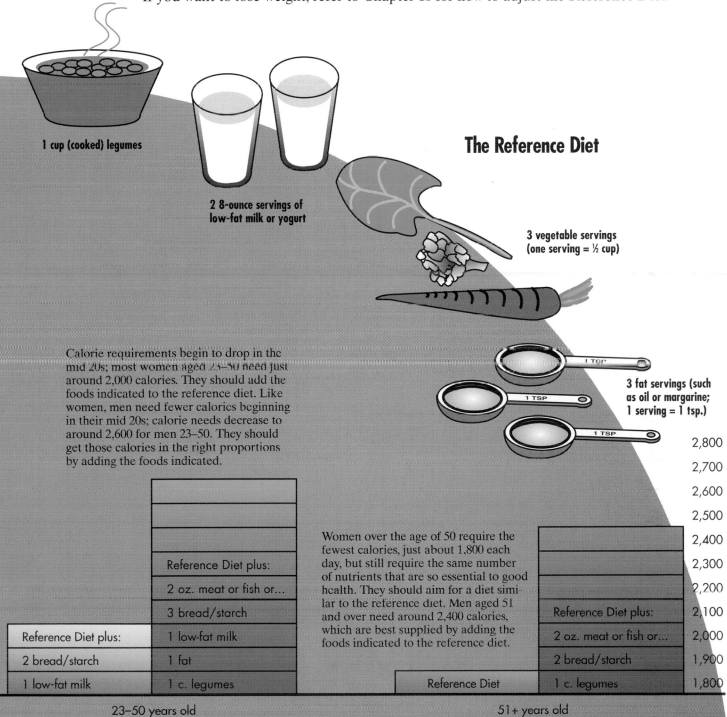

1 cup (cooked) legumes

The Reference Diet

2 8-ounce servings of low-fat milk or yogurt

3 vegetable servings (one serving = ½ cup)

3 fat servings (such as oil or margarine; 1 serving = 1 tsp.)

Calorie requirements begin to drop in the mid 20s; most women aged 23–50 need just around 2,000 calories. They should add the foods indicated to the reference diet. Like women, men need fewer calories beginning in their mid 20s; calorie needs decrease to around 2,600 for men 23–50. They should get those calories in the right proportions by adding the foods indicated.

Women over the age of 50 require the fewest calories, just about 1,800 each day, but still require the same number of nutrients that are so essential to good health. They should aim for a diet similar to the reference diet. Men aged 51 and over need around 2,400 calories, which are best supplied by adding the foods indicated to the reference diet.

	Reference Diet plus:	2,800
		2,700
		2,600
		2,500
		2,400
Reference Diet plus:		2,300
2 oz. meat or fish or...		2,200
3 bread/starch	Reference Diet plus:	2,100
Reference Diet plus:	1 low-fat milk	2 oz. meat or fish or...	2,000
2 bread/starch	1 fat	2 bread/starch	1,900
1 low-fat milk	1 c. legumes	Reference Diet	1 c. legumes	1,800

23–50 years old

51+ years old

How to Get Protein without Excess Fat

All protein foods, including those of animal and vegetable origin, can and *should* be part of a healthy diet. There are three keys to lightening up your protein foods: choosing leaner cuts of meat, limiting portion size, and preparing food to make it as lowfat as possible. In a week's time, plan meals so that by the end of the week you've had each type of protein food: beef, pork, poultry, fish, cheese, and grains or legumes. Try to choose grains and legumes two nights of the week, or, if they don't strike your fancy, weekly alternate a second meal of what you do enjoy.

There are three keys to eating leaner beef. The cut: "Round" and "loin" cuts of beef are the leanest. The grade: Beef is graded by the United States Department of Agriculture (USDA). The "select" grade contains the least amount of marbling, or flecks of fat in it. "Choice" beef is the second leanest grade of beef. The preparation: First trim all visible fat, and then roast, broil, or grill, without added fat. Compare the fat content of the three-ounce portions of cooked beef shown here.

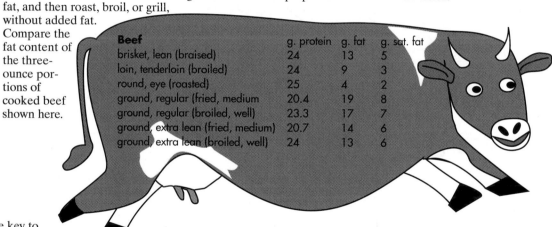

Beef	g. protein	g. fat	g. sat. fat
brisket, lean (braised)	24	13	5
loin, tenderloin (broiled)	24	9	3
round, eye (roasted)	25	4	2
ground, regular (fried, medium	20.4	19	8
ground, regular (broiled, well)	23.3	17	7
ground, extra lean (fried, medium)	20.7	14	6
ground, extra lean (broiled, well)	24	13	6

Portion Size The key to fat control is choosing lower-fat cuts of meat and poultry, but this works only if you also watch your portions. Most Americans (except women) eat far too much protein. Your meat serving should be about the size of a standard deck of playing cards, including the depth of that deck of cards. Put another way, it's the size that'll fit into your palm.

Prepared correctly, fish is an excellent source of lean protein, and also of omega-3 fatty acids (which are thought to protect against heart disease). Check out the fat content of the following 3-ounce portions of fish. Note that you shouldn't bother to choose a fish sandwich in a fast food establishment if what you really want is a hamburger!

Fish & Shellfish	g. protein	g. fat	g. sat. fat
cod (baked or broiled)	19.4	0.7	0.1
Alaska king crab	16.5	1.3	0.1
fish fillets (frozen) batter dipped	8	13	2.6
grouper	21	1.1	0.3
lobster	17.4	0.5	0.1
tuna, canned in oil	24.8	7.0	1.3
tuna, canned in water	21.7	0.7	0.2
fast food fish sandwich	20	25	4
shrimp	17.8	0.9	0.2
salmon, Atlantic	21.6	6.9	1.1

Cheese is an excellent source of protein that also boosts your calcium intake. By nature, cheeses are loaded with fat, but many of the lower-fat varieties make great substitutes. Here are some examples of how you can cut the fat by using lower-fat substitutes (all calculated for 3-ounce portions).

Cheese	g. protein	g. fat	g. sat. fat
cheddar, regular	21	28.2	18
cheddar, lowfat	21	6	4
mozzarella, regular	16	18.4	11
mozzarella, part-skim	23	14.5	9
ricotta, regular	9	11	7
ricotta, part-skim	9.6	6.7	4
ricotta, fat-free	9.6	0	0
cottage, small curd	10.7	3.8	2.4
cottage, 2% fat	11.7	1.6	1
cottage, fat-free	11.7	0	0

Grains & Legumes	g. protein	g. fat	g. sat. fat
lentils, 1 c. cooked	18	0.7	0.1
corn, 1 c.	5	2.2	0.4
brown rice, 1 c.	4.5	1.6	0.3
kidney beans, 1 c.	15.4	0.9	0.1
lima beans, 1 c. (add to corn)	14.7	0.7	0.2
chick peas, 1 c. (add cornbread)	14.5	4.3	0.4

Combined correctly, grains and legumes can give you a complete source of protein with very little fat. Here are some examples of how much protein you can get and the minimal fat charge incurred (grouped in combinations to yield complete proteins).

Chicken and turkey add great variety to your protein repertoire, but be sure to trim the fat, skin the meat, and cook it without added fat. Compare the following 3-ounce portions.

Chicken	g. protein	g. fat	g. sat. fat
breast w/skin (batter fried)	31.2	7.3	2
breast no skin (roasted)	26.7	3.1	0.9
breast fast food (fried)	33	22.3	5.5
chicken sandwich fast food	26	40	8
Turkey (roasted)			
light meat no skin	25.6	2.7	0.8
light meat w/skin	24.5	7.1	2
dark meat no skin	24.5	6.1	2
dark meat w/skin	23.5	9.8	3

Grains & Legumes	g. protein	g. fat	g. sat. fat
corn tortilla, large	2.1	1.1	0
pinto beans, 1 c.	14	0.9	0.2
rice cakes, two	1	0	0
peanut butter, 2 tbsp.	7.0	16	3.1
navy beans, 1 c.	15.8	1.0	0.3
rye bread, 2 slices	4.2	2	0
bulgur, 1 c.	5.6	0.4	0.1
red lentils, ½ c.	9	0.4	0

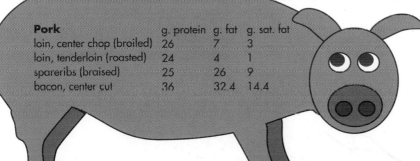

Pork	g. protein	g. fat	g. sat. fat
loin, center chop (broiled)	26	7	3
loin, tenderloin (roasted)	24	4	1
spareribs (braised)	25	26	9
bacon, center cut	36	32.4	14.4

Contrary to popular belief, pork can be part of a lower-fat, healthy-heart diet. The trick is in how you pick the cuts (pork is not graded), and how you cook it. The cut: Go for loin and leg cuts, the leanest around. Prepare pork by broiling, baking, or grilling without any added fat. Check for yourself (all 3 ounces, cooked and trimmed).

How to Get Carbohydrates without Excess Fat

There's no doubt about it: Complex carbohydrates are the best source of fuel for all bodies (and they're loaded with plenty of nutrients, too!). Try to get your carbohydrates close to the way they're found in nature. Remember: The more refined and processed they are, the fewer nutrients and more fat they probably have. You can choose lower-fat carbohydrates any time of the day. Here's how.

At breakfast, go for whole-grain bagels, breads, and cereals. Watch out for hidden fat mines in unsuspected sources.

Bread	g. fat	g. sat. fat
cracked wheat, 1 oz.	0.9	0
bagel, whole wheat	0.8	0.1
w/2 tbsp:		
cream cheese	11	6.5
nonfat cream cheese	0.8	0.1
jam	0.9	0.1
oatmeal, 1 c.	2.3	0.4
French cruller	10.4	2.7
croissant	12	6.7
blueberry muffin	7.4	1.4
granola, 1 c.	33.2	5.8

Cracker (1 oz.)	g. fat	g. sat. fat
fat-free, any type	0	0
saltines	3.4	0.6
100% stoned wheat	3.9	1.2
oat thins	3.4	0.6
cheese	7.1	2.7
round buttery	7.2	1.4
thin wheat	6.3	2.5
cheese filled	6	1.6

Vegetable soup and rice or pasta for lunch? Choose carefully, especially the crackers to accompany the soup!

Rice & Pasta (1 c.)	g. fat	g. sat. fat
brown rice	1.8	1.4
flavored rice, box mix	8.8	1.8
pasta	0.9	0.1
pasta primavera, box mix	10.4	3

Grazing for a midafternoon snack? Head for the whole-wheat pretzels or air-popped popcorn.

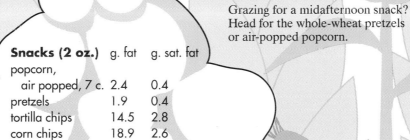

Snacks (2 oz.)	g. fat	g. sat. fat
popcorn,		
air popped, 7 c.	2.4	0.4
pretzels	1.9	0.4
tortilla chips	14.5	2.8
corn chips	18.9	2.6
potato chips	19.6	6.2

Potato	g. fat	g. sat. fat
baked w/skin	0.2	0
w/2 tbsp:		
nonfat sour cream	0.2	0
sour cream	6.2	3.8
potato salad, 1 c.	14.4	2.1
French fries, 3 oz.	14.1	5.8
au gratin, box, 1 c.	10	6.4

Potatoes complete any dinner, but eat them as they are plucked from the earth. See what happens as you change them and smother them.

Hankering for a little something after dinner? Choose carefully, or wait until you've hit your special dessert night to splurge!

Dessert	g. fat	g. sat. fat
angel food cake, slice	0.4	0
pound cake, slice	5.8	3.2
sugar cookie, 2 oz.	12	3.1
chocolate, 1 oz.	8.7	5.2
cheesecake, slice	20.7	10.6
shortcake, slice	12.1	3.2

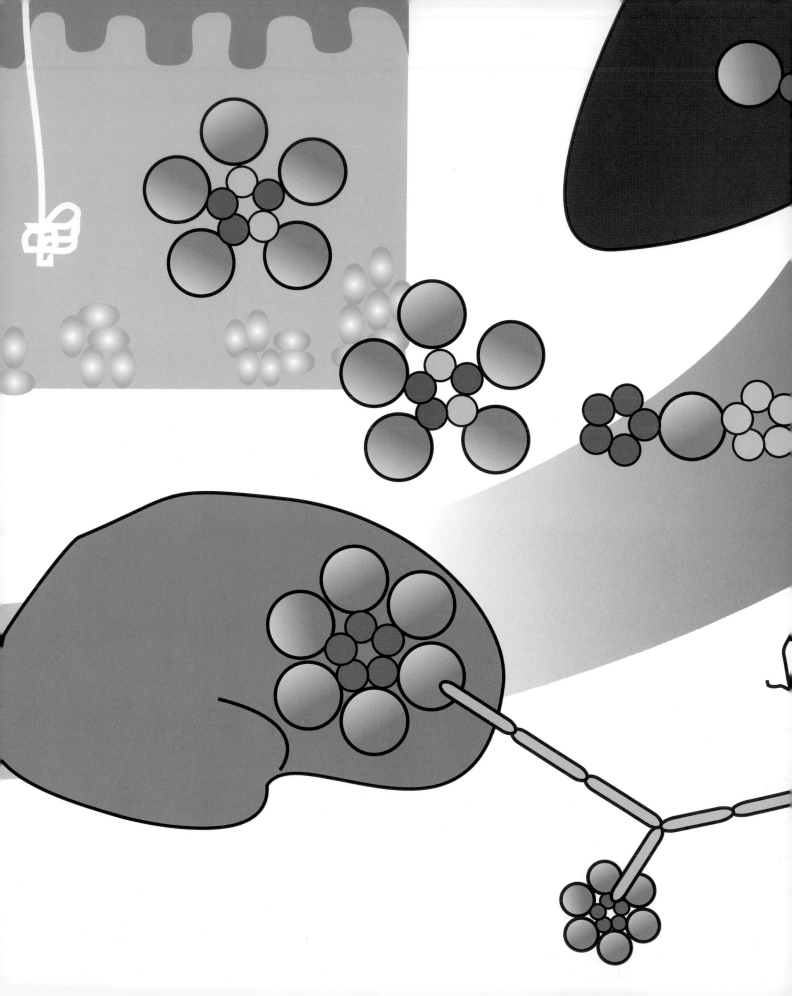

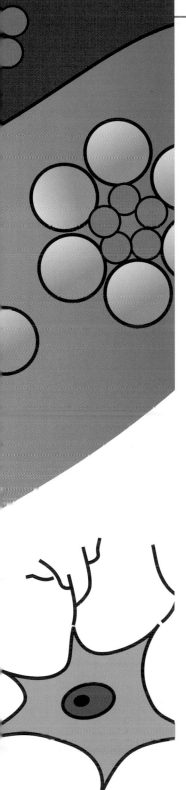

MICRONUTRIENTS: THE FINER DETAILS OF GREAT HEALTH

CONTENTS

Chapter 5   Fat-Soluble Vitamins: They Stick to Your Ribs
48

Chapter 6   Water-Soluble Vitamins
56

Chapter 7   Vitamins as Antioxidants: Radical Protection
64

Chapter 8   Minerals: Lending Strength and Glow
to Good Health
70

Chapter 9   Calcium: More Than Strong Bones
80

NOW THAT YOU know how to divide your calories among the macronutrients—carbohydrate, fat, and protein—you're ready to learn the finer details of good nutrition. Getting enough calories and protein simply isn't enough: The body craves literally dozens of vitamins and minerals to digest, absorb, and metabolize those calories, to grow, to heal injuries, to fight disease, and to drive the thousands of chemical reactions taking place in the body every second. Think of the macronutrients as the bricks from which the body is made and the mix of micronutrients as the cement holding them together.

It's a rare nutrient that works alone to accomplish a task—most work in concert with others. For example, calcium, vitamin A, phosphorus, fluoride, copper, and manganese are all necessary to form bone tissue. Red blood cells need at least iron, vitamin C, copper, B-6, B-12, and riboflavin.

A plethora of research has identified the amounts of nutrients we need for good health, values called Recommended Dietary Allowances, or RDAs. These values are set with a generous margin of safety (for healthy people); in other words, experts set a level slightly higher than you actually need. Think of that extra amount as a safety net for occasional times of increased need.

Many Americans, recognizing the critical importance of micronutrients, are jumping on the vitamin supplement bandwagon—and carrying a good thing too far. Vitamin and mineral enthusiasts are investing a virtual fortune in supplements, popping one or several pills daily.

This overzealous enthusiasm can be downright dangerous. As you'll read in this section, consuming more than the RDA can cause toxic side effects, or interfere with the absorption or metabolism of other nutrients. For some vitamins and minerals, amounts many, many times the RDA are necessary to cause undesirable side effects, but sometimes levels just slightly higher than the RDA are dangerous.

Overconsuming vitamins and minerals is also expensive. Americans spend billions of dollars a year on supplements, most of it money down the drain.

There's another problem with getting your nutrients from pills instead of food. Nutrition is a relatively new science, with the first nutrients identified just at the turn of the century. In fact, scientists are still discovering factors in food that are essential to disease prevention and a healthier body. They are also discovering important new information about factors they thought they knew—vitamins, for example. What's more, many nutrition experts agree that there are, no doubt, still-unidentified substances in food that are equally essential to life. In addition, there may be valuable naturally occurring combinations of nutrients in foods that we don't even know to try to imitate in pills. So, the next time you're tempted to grab a bottle of vitamin and mineral pills, take your dollars instead to the produce market and buy those pricey raspberries, mangoes, and red bell peppers that you might pass by because they're too expensive. You'll be far ahead nutritionally—with change left in your pocket.

PART TWO

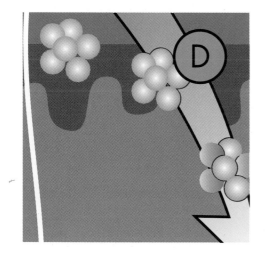

Fat-Soluble Vitamins: They Stick to Your Ribs

OF THE THIRTEEN vitamins our bodies need to function normally, four are known as *fat-soluble vitamins*. That's because they cannot be absorbed without the aid of dietary fat, and they're stored in fatty tissues and organs.

Why do we think of vitamins A, D, E, and K as vitamins that stick to our ribs? Because, unlike their water-soluble counterparts, excesses are not easily excreted. Instead, fat-soluble vitamins remain in the body until they are used. This translates into both good and bad news. Because they're stored in the body, you don't have to eat them every day to enjoy their benefits, and it's more difficult to run short of them. But this "stick-to-itness" also means that taking too much of these vitamins is more likely to cause trouble. Too much vitamin A or D is especially dangerous.

Fat-soluble vitamins come in different forms. Vitamin A, for example, is found as *retinol*, an already-formed vitamin, or as *carotenoids*, forms that are converted to vitamin A by the body. One of these, *beta-carotene*, has received considerable press for its role as an antioxidant. While the most exciting news about fat-soluble vitamins concerns their antioxidant capabilities, they have other crucial roles. This chapter focuses on these more traditional jobs; Chapter 7 explains their antioxidant role.

Vitamin A   Many people think orange when they think of vitamin A. That's because the carotenoids, substances that turn into vitamin A in the body, lend an orange-yellow color to some fruits and vegetables. But not all carotenoids have vitamin A activity; some are simply pigments. And some foods, like dark green leafy vegetables, actually have lots of vitamin A–active carotenoids, but their pigments are overshadowed by others. That means you can't rely on orange color alone to help you choose vitamin A–rich foods.

Do you remember your mother telling you to eat your carrots so you could see in the dark? Although many old tales about vitamins aren't true, this one is. Indeed, a critical function of vitamin A is to aid vision, especially in the dark. People who are deficient in vitamin A develop night blindness, or *nyctalopia*.

Vitamin A also keeps epithelial tissues healthy. Epithelium, which is the outermost layer of cells on surfaces inside and outside the body, lines the mucous membranes of the nose. It also lines the eye, the gastrointestinal, respiratory, and genitourinary tracts, and forms the outer-most layer of skin.

A lack of vitamin A weakens epithelial tissues, making them more susceptible to invasion by germs, which can lead to infection. Vitamin A deficiency may also lead to diseases of the gastrointestinal, respiratory, and genitourinary systems; some evidence indicates such weakened tissues are more susceptible to cancer. Emerging evidence, in fact, links a lack of vitamin A to cervical cancer. Some researchers are testing a vita-min A cream for its ability to prevent cervical cancer, and other research probes vita-min A's ability to prevent precancerous mouth lesions common in smokers and users of smokeless tobacco. Vitamin A is also essential to normal bone growth and fetal de-velopment and is even a necessary ingredient in successful breast-feeding.

But while some is absolutely necessary to life and good health, getting too much vitamin A can be very dangerous. Symptoms of toxicity include fatigue, severe headaches, blurred vision, insomnia, loss of body hair, menstrual irregularities, skin rashes, and joint pain; at extreme doses, there can be liver and brain damage. If you're an adult female, you need 800 micrograms (or ½ carrot). Males should aim for 1,000 micrograms. Getting just 10 times the RDA (of Vitamin A, not its carotenoid precur-sor) for any length of time can lead to toxicity.

Vitamin D: Healthy Bones and More   Vitamin D is best known for its pivotal role in building strong bones. In fact, it is the single most important substance in help-ing the body absorb and use calcium.

But vitamin D is essential to good health for other reasons, too. There is emerging evidence that it reduces the risk of colon cancer, and other research focuses on its abil-ity to *treat* cancer. Animal studies also reveal vitamin D's crucial role in normal fetal development.

Fortunately, most of the vitamin D we need can be manufactured in the skin with the sun's aid. Through a fascinating chemical process, a form of cholesterol found under the skin is transformed into vitamin D. Just 10–20 minutes of sun exposure (to the face and hands) three times per week makes enough vitamin D. People with darker skin and the elderly, though, have a decreased ability to manufacture vitamin D and should turn to dietary sources of vitamin D (as should people who don't have sufficient sun exposure—which can be true for everyone in the winter).

As with vitamin A, too much vitamin D can be dangerous, and the danger arises at doses just five times over the adult RDA of 200 international units (I.U.). Getting too much vitamin D causes excess calcium to circulate in the blood and subsequently become deposited in soft tissues—leading to kidney and heart damage. (It's worth noting that sun exposure plus milk should not result in a vitamin D overdose.) When you think of vitamins A and D, remember that while some is absolutely necessary, more is definitely not better!

Vitamin E Did someone ever tell you to rub the contents of a vitamin E capsule into your skin, either to heal a wound or keep skin healthy? Unfortunately, such advice is probably unfounded (although the oil coats the skin, preventing moisture loss, but any type of oil can do this job). But vitamin E is essential to good health for other reasons.

Vitamin E is a well-known guardian of healthy tissues. It maintains tissue integrity, basically by not allowing the fatty component of tissues to become rancid (think of rancidity as similar to the process by which metal rusts). In a similar process, vitamin E keeps red blood cells strong. Not getting enough vitamin E can result in breakdown of red blood cells and, eventually, anemia.

Although there is not conclusive evidence, most experts think that vitamin E is relatively nontoxic, even at doses many times the RDA, which is 8 I.U. for women and 10 I.U. for men.

Interestingly, eating too much polyunsaturated fat increases the body's requirement for vitamin E—yet another reason to keep fat intake down to a healthy level!

Vitamin K We hear the least about vitamin K, and for good reason. Although vitamin K's role is no less important than any other vitamin's—it's needed to make blood clot, to build strong bones (especially in the elderly), and for healthy kidney tissues—we don't usually need to worry about getting enough of it. Bacteria that normally live in the intestinal tract make 80% of the vitamin K we need (adults need between 60 and 80 micrograms of vitamin K a day). In some cases, infants may not have the bacteria necessary to manufacture vitamin K, and people taking antibiotics may temporarily lose their ability to make enough vitamin K. Overall, we still need to get some vitamin K from a healthy diet. Like large amounts of vitamin E, large amounts of dietary vitamin K do not appear to cause serious harm.

Refer to the following pages to help you factor in the right foods to harvest all essential fat-soluble vitamins.

How the Body Gets Fat-Soluble Vitamins

Because the fat-soluble vitamins A, D, E, and K are found in a wide variety of foods, they're easy to get. Here are some foods high in each of these vitamins, and how much you need to eat get your daily requirement (if you're an adult). Nature has also provided us another way to get vitamin D: the sun. Exposing your face and hands to just 10 to 20 minutes of sunshine three times a week ensures that you'll meet your daily quota. Check out the following foods high in fat-soluble vitamins.

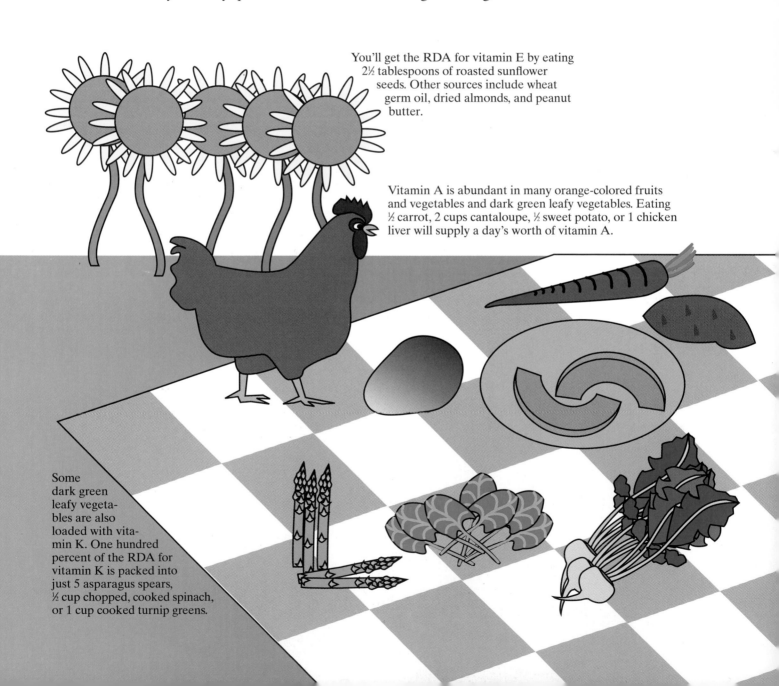

You'll get the RDA for vitamin E by eating 2½ tablespoons of roasted sunflower seeds. Other sources include wheat germ oil, dried almonds, and peanut butter.

Vitamin A is abundant in many orange-colored fruits and vegetables and dark green leafy vegetables. Eating ½ carrot, 2 cups cantaloupe, ½ sweet potato, or 1 chicken liver will supply a day's worth of vitamin A.

Some dark green leafy vegetables are also loaded with vitamin K. One hundred percent of the RDA for vitamin K is packed into just 5 asparagus spears, ½ cup chopped, cooked spinach, or 1 cup cooked turnip greens.

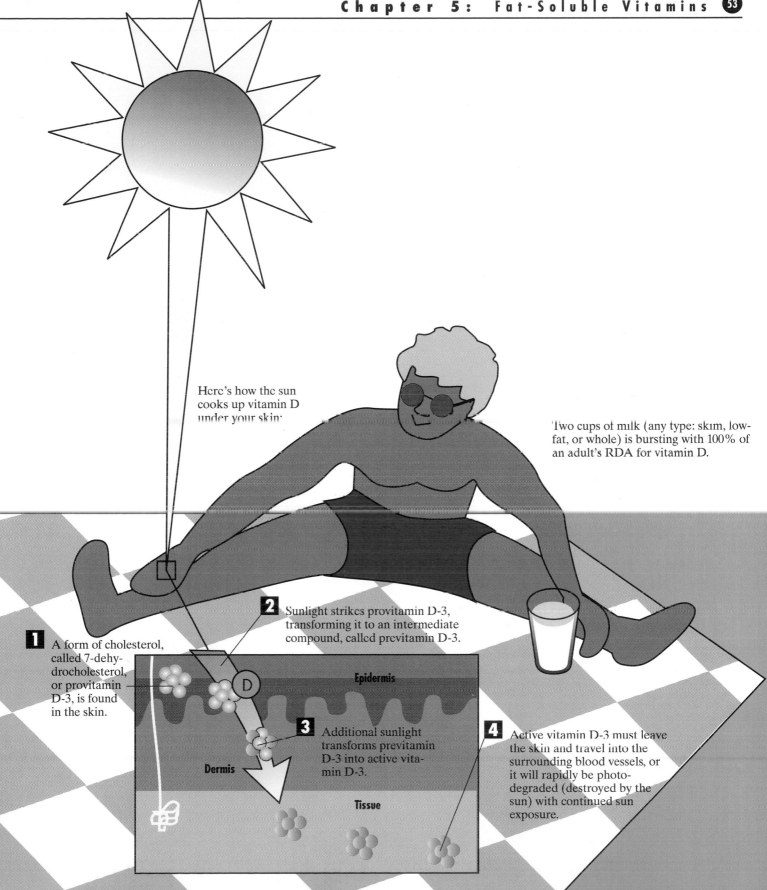

Here's how the sun cooks up vitamin D under your skin:

Two cups of milk (any type: skim, low-fat, or whole) is bursting with 100% of an adult's RDA for vitamin D.

1 A form of cholesterol, called 7-dehy-drocholesterol, or provitamin D-3, is found in the skin.

2 Sunlight strikes provitamin D-3, transforming it to an intermediate compound, called previtamin D-3.

3 Additional sunlight transforms previtamin D-3 into active vitamin D-3.

4 Active vitamin D-3 must leave the skin and travel into the surrounding blood vessels, or it will rapidly be photo-degraded (destroyed by the sun) with continued sun exposure.

Epidermis

Dermis

Tissue

What the Body Does with Vitamin D

While the body does not tolerate an overdose of most nutrients, it is especially intolerant of too much of the fat-soluble vitamins A and D. Here, for example, is what the body does with too much—and also too little and the right amount—of vitamin D.

1 Vitamin D is necessary for the absorption of calcium and phosphorus, two of the minerals essential to form and maintain strong bones.

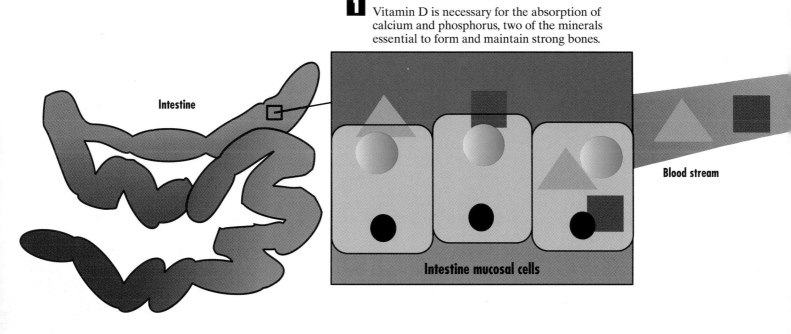

Intestine

Intestine mucosal cells

Blood stream

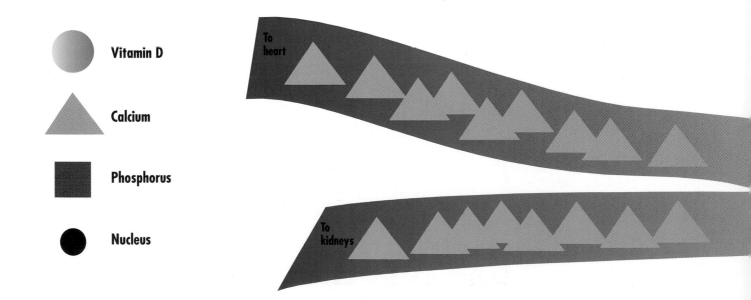

Vitamin D

Calcium

Phosphorus

Nucleus

To heart

To kidneys

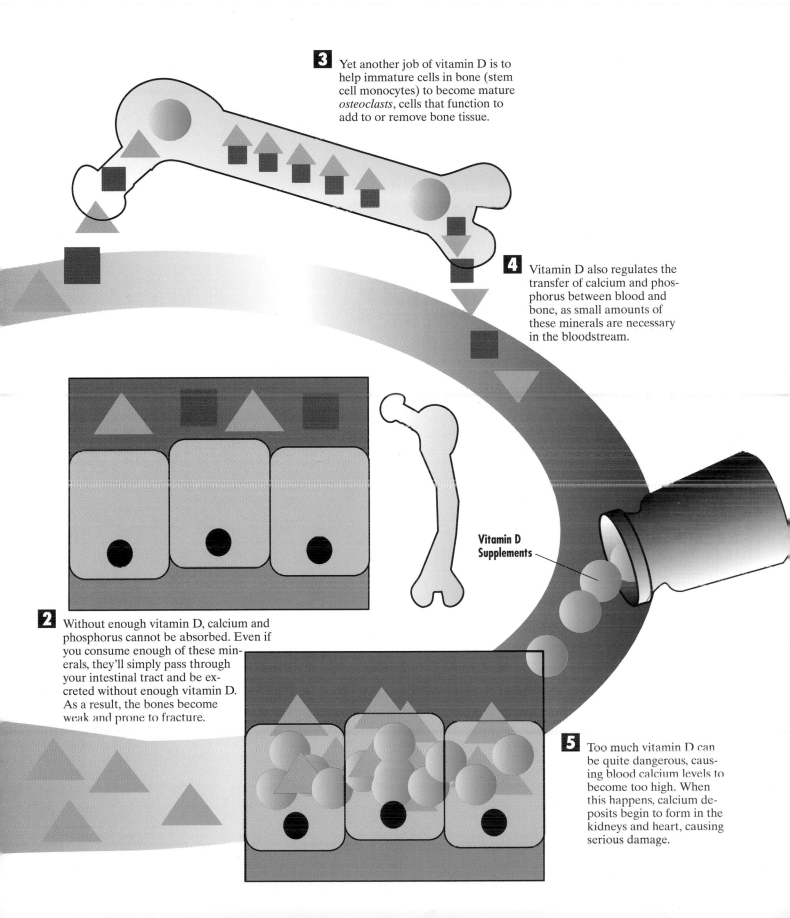

3 Yet another job of vitamin D is to help immature cells in bone (stem cell monocytes) to become mature *osteoclasts*, cells that function to add to or remove bone tissue.

4 Vitamin D also regulates the transfer of calcium and phosphorus between blood and bone, as small amounts of these minerals are necessary in the bloodstream.

Vitamin D Supplements

2 Without enough vitamin D, calcium and phosphorus cannot be absorbed. Even if you consume enough of these minerals, they'll simply pass through your intestinal tract and be excreted without enough vitamin D. As a result, the bones become weak and prone to fracture.

5 Too much vitamin D can be quite dangerous, causing blood calcium levels to become too high. When this happens, calcium deposits begin to form in the kidneys and heart, causing serious damage.

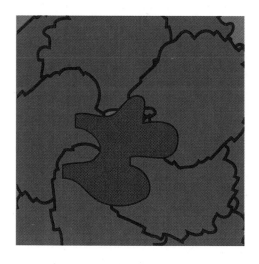

CHAPTER 6

Water-Soluble Vitamins

CONSIDERING THAT THE first vitamin was discovered less than 100 years ago, it's no surprise that scientists are still uncovering their life-sustaining mysteries. While we've known, for example, that folic acid helps prevent a certain type of anemia, it's just within the past couple of years that scientists have discovered folic acid's quintessential role in preventing a birth defect called spina bifida and in preventing cancer and heart disease. Similarly, vitamins B-6 and B-12 are now recognized for their role in staving off heart disease and niacin for its ability to lower blood cholesterol.

If there ever is a magic bullet for achieving the highest level of good health, it will be packed full of the water-soluble vitamins. There are nine of them: C, B-1 (thiamin), B-2 (riboflavin), B-3 (niacin), B-6 (pyridoxine), B-12 (cobalamin), folic acid, pantothenic acid, and biotin. Every single one contributes significantly to our health—not one is optional or even "just a little" important, nor can one substitute for another.

Consider this analogy: If you leave out baking powder when baking a cake, the cake tastes fine, but it looks like a pancake. If you omit half the sugar, flavor is compromised. Every single ingredient, in just the right amount, is necessary to make the best-tasting and best-looking cake. So it is with vitamins and your health.

Alarmingly, certain water-soluble vitamins are the most underconsumed nutrients in the United States. Surveys reveal that many Americans are deficient in B-6, folic acid, riboflavin, and C. Why? As we get busier, we turn increasingly to fast and precooked meals, often highly refined (made of nutrient-poor white flour, rather than nutrient-packed whole grains) and lacking in fresh produce. Even when eating a home-cooked meal, many people don't take the time to prepare whole-grain, fruit, and vegetable dishes.

For example, if you're the average adult trying to eat a healthy diet, you might grab a cup of coffee and plain bagel on the way to work; a hamburger and diet cola at lunch; frozen low fat yogurt in the afternoon; heat a frozen macaroni and cheese entree and team it with an iceberg lettuce salad at dinner; and later snack on apples and popcorn. Even though you've managed to eat a healthy calorie level, you will come up short on every single water-soluble vitamin—getting less than one-quarter of the recommended amounts of vitamin C and B-6, and just about half of most others.

Water-soluble vitamins get their name because they dissolve into the watery fluids of our body. Because of this, we don't store them, which means the following: It's more difficult to experience toxic side-effects; it's easier to experience deficiencies (we have to eat them regularly to avoid coming up short); and they're more fragile (they're more easily destroyed during cooking and storage).

Here's a quick rundown of the most important jobs each nutrient performs. Refer to the following pages for more detailed information on how to load up your magic bullet with Bs and C.

B-1 (Thiamin)   Without thiamin, you couldn't burn carbohydrates to fuel your body. Unfortunately, many people mistakenly think large quantities of thiamin (and other B-vitamins) will supply extra energy, but it doesn't work that way. (Another analogy helps clarify the point: Just as you cannot put extra gas in your car to make it go farther because the excess runs out of the gas tank, water-soluble vitamins over the amount our bodies can use are simply excreted.) Thiamin also plays a very specialized role in keeping brain, nerve, and heart cells healthy.

B-2 (Riboflavin)   Without riboflavin, you couldn't unlock the energy found in carbohydrates (even if you had enough thiamin), nor could you form healthy red blood cells. In addition, you might have dry, scaly skin and your eyes would be sensitive to light. This vitamin is especially sensitive to heat and light, which means riboflavin-rich foods should be stored in the refrigerator or in the dark.

B-3 (Niacin)   Niacin is yet another key necessary for unlocking carbohydrates' energy. It has several other roles, including keeping our skin, nerves, and digestive system healthy. Very large doses of niacin may help lower LDL, or bad cholesterol, and raise HDL, or good cholesterol, thereby helping to stave off heart disease. But at the doses necessary to achieve this benefit—1,000 milligrams versus the required 15–19 milligrams—it is considered a medication and not a vitamin. Only take such quantities with your physician's recommendation. Taking large doses of niacin for any period of time can lead to liver damage, ulcers, abnormally high blood sugar, itching, and flushed complexion.

B-6 (Pyroxidine)   B-6 is to protein what B-1, B-2, and B-3 are to carbohydrates: It's necessary for breaking down protein. It's also needed to make nonessential amino acids and is an essential component of red blood cells, antibodies (infection fighters), and insulin. Some studies suggest that taking large doses of B-6 relieves premenstrual syndrome for for some women. But such doses can lead to serious neurological problems and are not recommended.

Folic Acid (Folacin)   One of this century's greatest scientific discoveries is that folic acid can prevent spina bifida and related birth defects. Now, researchers find it may also lower heart disease and cancer risk. Traditionally, folic acid has been known for working in concert with B-12 to make healthy red blood cells and for decoding genetic information to make new cells and tissues.

In 1989, experts recommended a lower RDA for folic acid, dropping the recommendation from 400 mcg to 200 mcg for men and 180 mcg for women. But research has shown that folic acid's ability to prevent heart disease is impaired at even 280 mcg per day. Some experts, therefore, recommend we raise the RDA back to 400 mcg for men and nonpregnant women, and to 800 mcg for pregnant women. Currently, all women of child-bearing age are advised to get 400 mcg per day. (Because most women don't even know they're pregnant until after the changes leading to spina bifida occur, the U.S. Public Health Service recommends the higher level for all women who could potentially become pregnant.) Don't go overboard, though, as too much folic acid can mask the symptoms of B-12 deficiency, which can cause permanent nerve damage.

B-12 (Cobalamin)   Like folic acid, B-12 helps decode genetic information to manufacture new cells and is an important ingredient in red blood cell formation. It also helps keep the nervous system healthy. B-12 is found almost exclusively in foods of animal origin. Unlike other water-soluble vitamins, B-12 needs help to be absorbed. Intrinsic factor, made by the lining of the stomach, shuttles B-12 into cells. People with stomach troubles (especially the elderly) may not be able to absorb enough B-12, and they may need B-12 injections (but people who absorb B-12 normally do not benefit from B-12 shots). B-12 deficiency causes pernicious anemia, a disease that also includes serious nervous system abnormalities.

Pantothenic Acid and Biotin   Although we know they're essential to good health, there isn't an RDA for these two B-vitamins. That's because they occur so widely in foods and also because a deficiency has never been observed.

Vitamin C   Many people think vitamin C prevents or cures colds. But 20 years of research has failed to prove this claim. Still, vitamin C is critically important to good health: It helps the body to build healthy bones, teeth, skin, and tendons; to absorb iron; to heal wounds; and to resist infections. Cigarette smokers use up their vitamin C much more rapidly than nonsmokers and therefore need about 50% more. Vitamin C is now thought of as one of the antioxidant nutrients (see Chapter 7). Taking excessive vitamin C may cause diarrhea and may also change the results of certain medical tests.

Water-Soluble Vitamins: Absorbed, Excreted, but Not Stored

Some of these essential nutrients are found in fruits and vegetables, some in grains, some in dairy products, some in legumes, and some in meat, and many are found in more than one source. That's why it's important to eat a balanced diet—one that contains lots of different foods from all the major food groups. And because they're not stored, it's critically important to consume the right amounts daily.

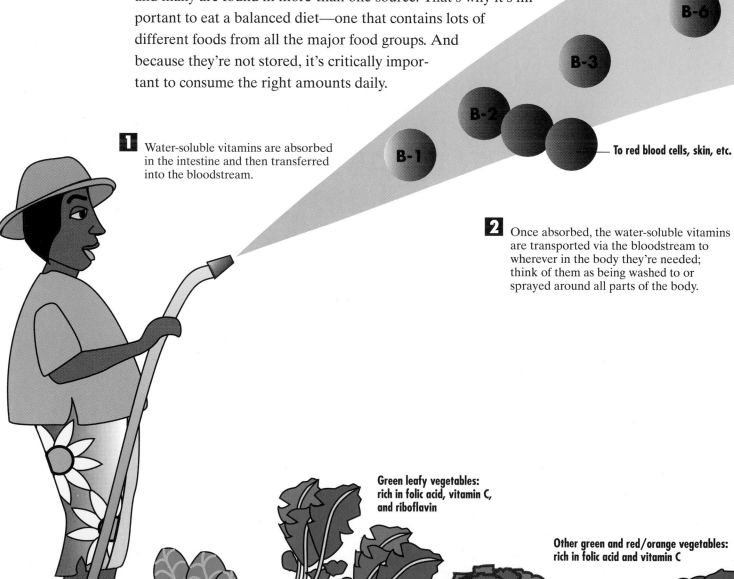

B-6

B-3

B-2

B-1

— To red blood cells, skin, etc.

1 Water-soluble vitamins are absorbed in the intestine and then transferred into the bloodstream.

2 Once absorbed, the water-soluble vitamins are transported via the bloodstream to wherever in the body they're needed; think of them as being washed to or sprayed around all parts of the body.

Green leafy vegetables: rich in folic acid, vitamin C, and riboflavin

Other green and red/orange vegetables: rich in folic acid and vitamin C

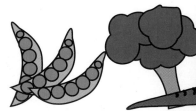

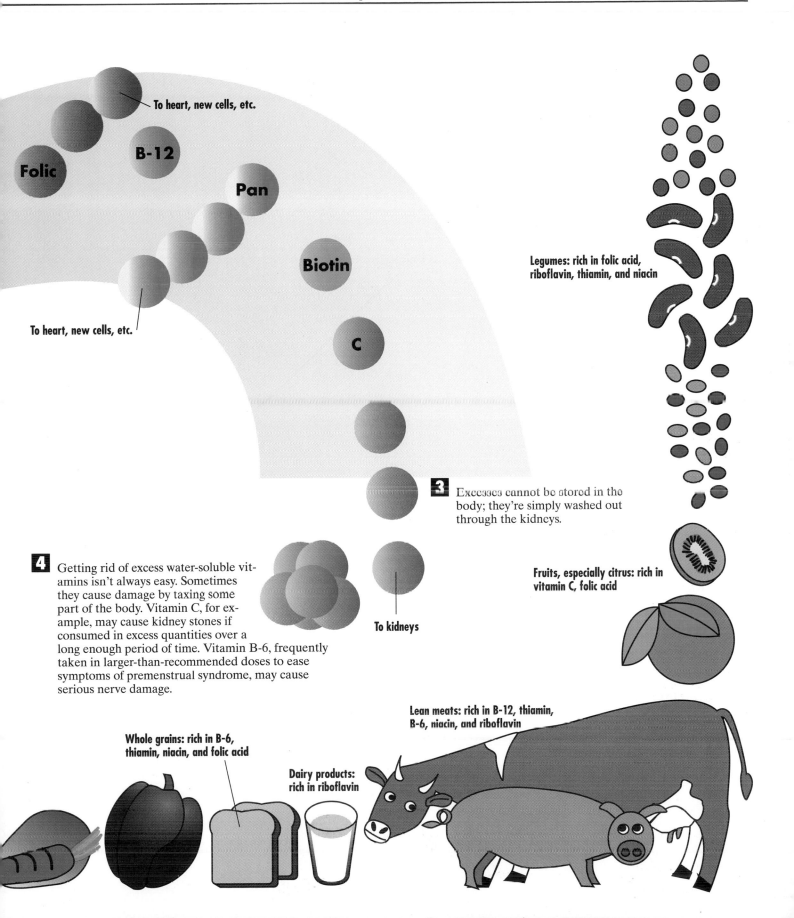

To heart, new cells, etc.

B-12

Folic

Pan

Biotin

C

To heart, new cells, etc.

Legumes: rich in folic acid, riboflavin, thiamin, and niacin

3 Excesses cannot be stored in the body; they're simply washed out through the kidneys.

4 Getting rid of excess water-soluble vitamins isn't always easy. Sometimes they cause damage by taxing some part of the body. Vitamin C, for example, may cause kidney stones if consumed in excess quantities over a long enough period of time. Vitamin B-6, frequently taken in larger-than-recommended doses to ease symptoms of premenstrual syndrome, may cause serious nerve damage.

To kidneys

Fruits, especially citrus: rich in vitamin C, folic acid

Lean meats: rich in B-12, thiamin, B-6, niacin, and riboflavin

Whole grains: rich in B-6, thiamin, niacin, and folic acid

Dairy products: rich in riboflavin

How the Body Uses Water-Soluble Vitamins: B-6 at Work

Each of the nine water-soluble vitamins is essential to great health. Not one is optional, nor can one substitute for another. Many work in concert with others to accomplish a task; for example, folic acid, B-12, B-6, and B-2 join forces to form and maintain healthy red blood cells. Here we see vitamin B-6 at work.

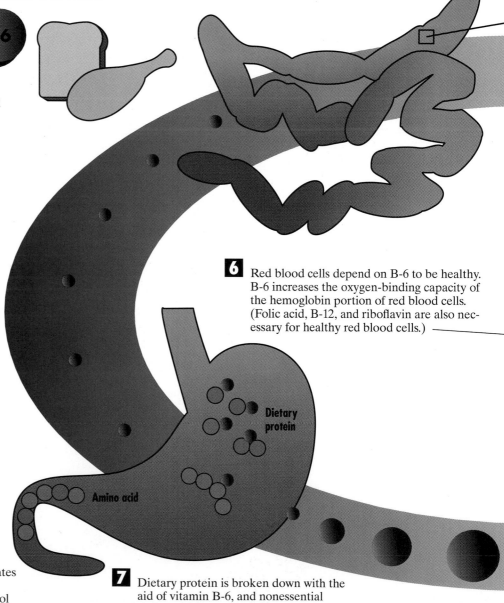

1 When we eat whole-grain foods and lean meats, we harvest lots of vitamin B-6. B-6 (pyroxidine) helps break down dietary protein and build nonessential amino acids in the body; it's an essential component of red blood cells, antibodies, and insulin.

B-1 (thiamin) unleashes energy from carbohydrates and keeps brain, nerve, and heart cells healthy.

B-2 (riboflavin) also works to unlock energy from carbohydrates, as well as keeping skin, eyes, and red blood cells healthy.

B-3 (niacin) unlocks energy from carbohydrates and keeps skin, nerves, and digestive system healthy; may help lower high blood cholesterol (but only under a doctor's supervision).

6 Red blood cells depend on B-6 to be healthy. B-6 increases the oxygen-binding capacity of the hemoglobin portion of red blood cells. (Folic acid, B-12, and riboflavin are also necessary for healthy red blood cells.)

Dietary protein

Amino acid

7 Dietary protein is broken down with the aid of vitamin B-6, and nonessential amino acids can only form inside the body with its help.

Folic

Folic acid prevents spina bifida and related birth defects (this has been heralded as one of the greatest medical discoveries of the decade); keeps red blood cells healthy, helps make new cells and tissues, and prevents cancer and heart disease.

2 Vitamin B-6 is absorbed in the small intestine. This form is not biologically active; in other words, the body must convert it to an active form.

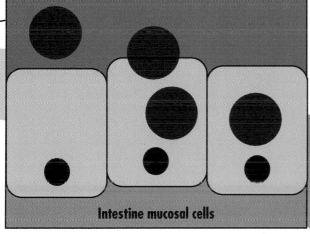

Intestine mucosal cells

B-12

B-12 (cobalamin) forms red blood cells and helps make new cells and tissues; keeps nervous system healthy.

3 Once absorbed, B-6 must be transported via the bloodstream to the liver. Inside the liver the inactive form of B-6 is converted into the active form. The active form of B-6 is then carried to many other parts of the body, where it is needed to catalyze or "start up" many chemical reactions or processes.

Pan

Pantothenic acid helps make and metabolize fats; forms hormones and cholesterol.

B-6

Biotin

Biotin helps form fatty acids and metabolize carbohydrates.

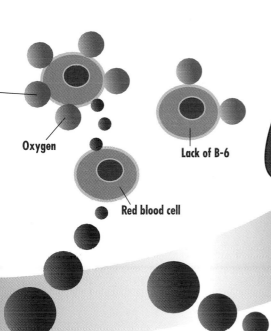

Oxygen

Lack of B-6

Red blood cell

C

Vitamin C helps build healthy bones, teeth, skin, and tendons; helps absorb iron; aids in wound healing; helps resist infections.

5 B-6 is also needed to keep cells in the nervous system healthy. (Thiamin, niacin, and B-12 also play a role in nerve-cell health.)

4 B-6 is needed to make *neurotransmitters*, brain chemicals that communicate important messages. Some of the neurotransmitters for which B-6 is an essential component are serotonin and norepinephrine.

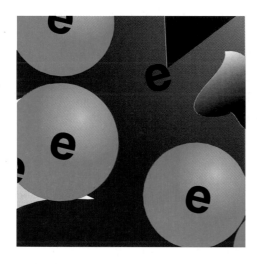

CHAPTER 7

Vitamins as Antioxidants: Radical Protection

SPEAKING OF NEW jobs for old vitamins, as we did in Chapter 6, three dietary substances have recently been recognized for their newly discovered role as guardians against heart disease and cancer, the two major killers in this country. Known as antioxidants, vitamins C and E and beta-carotene (a vitamin precursor) may well be the hottest dietary substances around. To achieve the potential disease-prevention benefits, doses much higher than the RDA of vitamins C and E are apparently needed, but exact amounts aren't yet known (there isn't an RDA for beta-carotene). Hordes of people are currently popping antioxidant supplements, hoping to stave off disease. However, although there is fairly convincing evidence that antioxidants are powerful adjuncts in preventing heart disease and cancer, you shouldn't head for the drug or health food store. Rather, it's best to try to get vitamin C and beta-carotene from food. Vitamin E is a little more complicated, as we'll see.

Why do we need antioxidants? Every cell in our body needs oxygen to generate energy. In the process of using that oxygen, by-products are formed, free radicals among them. A *free radical* is an atom that is missing an electron, which makes it unstable. In an attempt to stabilize itself, the free radical steals an electron from another atom. Each robbed atom, in turn, attempts to achieve stability, stealing an electron from a neighboring atom, thus creating a chain reaction.

Inside the body, free radicals steal electrons from cells, creating a chain reaction of cellular damage, or *oxidation*, as it's properly called. Oxidation is the same process by which metal rusts and butter turns rancid. In the body, oxidation contributes to the effects of aging, heart disease, cancer, cataracts, and infections.

Cells have a defensive strategy to disable free radicals and repair the damage they cause. And now research provides very compelling evidence that dietary antioxidants, vitamins A and C and beta-carotene, bolster this radical protection.

What is *not* known is the level of antioxidants necessary to confer radical protection, the best combination, and the side effects of taking the high doses that seem to be necessary. It *is* known that dietary antioxidants cannot undo damage caused by an unhealthy lifestyle. Someone who smokes, overeats, or doesn't exercise, for example, cannot take solace in popping antioxidant pills.

Also, it's best to get antioxidants from foods, rather than pills. Why? As you'll read in greater detail in Chapter 17, food contains nonnutritive substances—also recently discovered —that apparently play a role in cancer prevention and that cannot be produced in pill form. In addition, nutrition is a relatively new science, and there are no doubt other undiscovered substances in food that are essential to good health.

How do antioxidants work? Vitamin E is proving itself a fighter against heart disease. Researchers have known since the late 1980s that oxidized LDL cholesterol (bad cholesterol) is more likely to lodge in arteries. Once there, the oxidized LDLs lure white blood cells, which devour them. (Normally, white blood cells circulate in blood, policing our bodies for invading foreign substances—destroying bacteria and viruses, for example.) Over time, the LDL-engorged white cells expand within artery walls, narrowing the passageway. Research indicates that vitamin E may prevent LDL cholesterol from oxidizing and becoming so prone to lodging in arteries. How much vitamin E is necessary? Again, researchers haven't yet identified the exact number, but they suggest 100 international units (I.U.) to 400 I.U., which is significantly more than the RDA of 8 I.U. However, one study found that amounts over 100 I.U. conferred no additional benefit.

Let's take a look at the role of beta-carotene and vitamin C in fighting cancer. If the free-radical chain reaction causes extensive cell damage, cancer-causing changes may ensue. Antioxidants are thought to neutralize free radicals before such damage occurs. There's increasing evidence that dietary antioxidants, particularly beta-carotene, may prevent cervical cancer in women, lung cancer, skin cancer (especially in people with previous basal cell skin cancers), and colon cancer. Vitamin C may be particularly helpful in preventing stomach cancer; populations with typically low vitamin C intakes have higher rates of stomach cancer. Some researchers recommend that we increase vitamin C intake to 250 or even 1,000 milligrams daily (the RDA is just 60 milligrams), and that we aim for 6–30 milligrams of beta-carotene.

Vitamin C at antioxidant doses seems especially important in preventing cataracts. Cataracts occur when there is a change in the chemical composition of the eye's lens, and it's suspected that this change develops partly as a result of the oxidation of the protein that forms the lens.

Dietary antioxidants may delay some effects of aging, bringing people to their later years in much better health and with a younger appearance. Unimpeded, free radicals gradually chipping away at cells may exacerbate the formation of wrinkles, for example, and even the decline of the immune system.

Can high doses of antioxidants be dangerous? As we noted in Chapter 6, high doses of vitamin C may cause diarrhea and may change certain medical test results (in particular, blood sugar and fecal occult blood tests). It's still unclear, however, whether 1,000 milligrams is sufficient to cause such adverse effects; it's also unknown if getting 250 or 500 milligrams from food sources regularly has any negative effects at all.

Even fairly large doses of beta-carotene are apparently harmless. Although you may turn yellow or orange from eating a pound or two of carrots (which contain a large amount of beta-carotene) a day, you probably won't experience any other serious side effects. Not only is beta-carotene relatively nontoxic, but we're protected because the body controls the amount transformed into vitamin A, only making what it needs.

While research has failed to turn up evidence that a daily supplement of 400 I.U. vitamin E has negative side effects, few studies have followed people for more than 6 months or a year. The question of toxicity from long-term large doses remains largely unanswered. (It is known that people who take certain medication, including anticoagulants, may experience serious side effects from taking extra vitamin E; people with retinitis pigmentosa, a serious eye disease, may worsen that ailment.)

In the charts that follow, you'll find combinations of foods that supply antioxidant levels of vitamin C and beta-carotene, and 10–20 I.U. of vitamin E, as well as 400 micrograms of folic acid (it's included because it's found in many of the same foods as antioxidants). Yes, these suggestions probably include far more fruits and vegetables than you're accustomed to eating. But according to the National Cancer Institute, every American should eat 5 to 9 fruit and vegetable servings daily. Currently, just 23% of Americans say they eat 5 or more servings, and the majority eat just 1 or 2 servings. But if you add fruit to each meal, and one or two vegetables to both lunch and dinner, you're well on your way to a healthier life.

How Antioxidants Work

Dietary antioxidants may offer powerful protection against cancer, heart disease, cataracts, infection, and some effects of aging. Although experts don't know the exact amounts needed, recommendations range from 250–1,000 milligrams for vitamin C, 6–30 milligrams for beta carotene, and 100–400 I.U. for vitamin E. Try to get them from food instead of supplements (although it's hard to get that much vitamin E from food without blowing your calorie allowance). Here's how antioxidants work and how to get them in food.

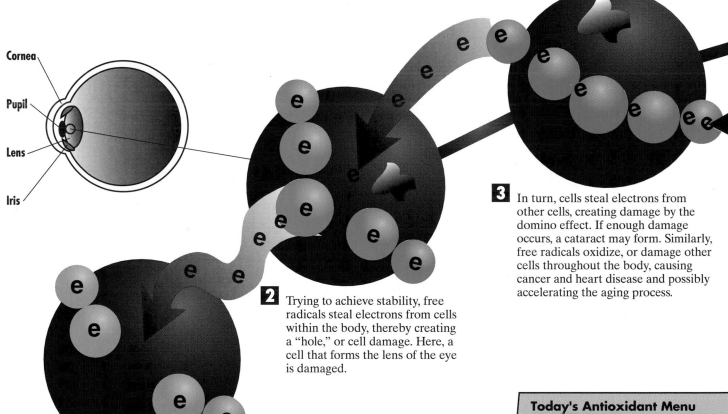

Cornea
Pupil
Lens
Iris

3 In turn, cells steal electrons from other cells, creating damage by the domino effect. If enough damage occurs, a cataract may form. Similarly, free radicals oxidize, or damage other cells throughout the body, causing cancer and heart disease and possibly accelerating the aging process.

2 Trying to achieve stability, free radicals steal electrons from cells within the body, thereby creating a "hole," or cell damage. Here, a cell that forms the lens of the eye is damaged.

1 Missing one electron, free radicals (formed as the body breaks down oxygen atoms) are unstable.

With this combination of foods, you'll get 500 milligrams vitamin C, 30–35 milligrams beta-carotene, and 10 I.U. vitamin E (you'll also get 400 micrograms folic acid; see Chapter 6). Just add in grains and protein for a complete diet!

Today's Antioxidant Menu
Breakfast
6 oz. orange juice
3 apricots
C
Lunch
Salad: ½ grated carrot,
½ c. chopped red pepper
1 chopped mango
½ c. raw spinach
Beta-carotene
Snack
6 oz. tomato juice
Dinner
1 c. cooked turnip greens
½ c. cooked cauliflower
E
Snack
1 orange

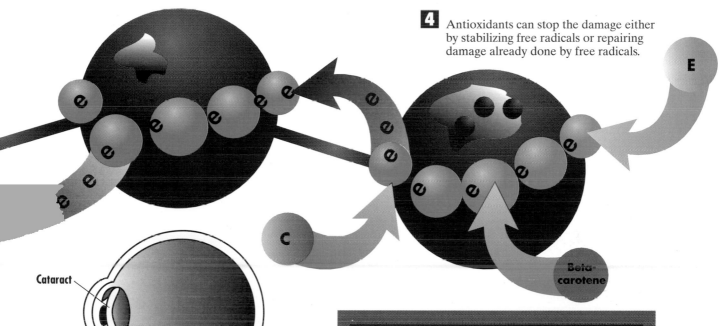

4 Antioxidants can stop the damage either by stabilizing free radicals or repairing damage already done by free radicals.

Cataract

Here's another combination of foods that gives you 500 milligrams of vitamin C, 30–35 milligrams beta-carotene, 10 I.U. vitamin E, and 400 micrograms folic acid.

Tomorrow's Antioxidant Menu
Breakfast
1 orange
Lunch
Salad: 1 grated carrot,
5 cherry tomatoes
1½ c. raw spinach
Snack
1 papaya
Dinner
½ c. cooked kale
5 brussels sprouts
1 slice watermelon
Snack
6 oz. cranberry juice
¼ c. peanuts

Antioxidant Hall of Fame

Top Beta-carotene Foods	mg.
½ c. canned pumpkin	27
1 baked sweet potato	25
1 carrot	20
1 c. cooked turnip greens	13
1 papaya	8.5
½ cantaloupe	8.6
½ c. cooked spinach	7.3

Top Vitamin C Foods	
1 papaya	187
½ c. chopped red pepper	95
1 c. strawberry slices	94
1 orange	80
6 oz. orange juice	66
5 brussel sprouts	65
1 mango	57

Top Vitamin E Foods	I.U.
¼ c. wheat germ	11
2 T. dry roasted sunflower seeds	8
1 c. cooked kale	7.4
1 sweet potato	5.4
1 papya	3.4
1 c. cooked turnip greens	2.8
1 mango	2.3

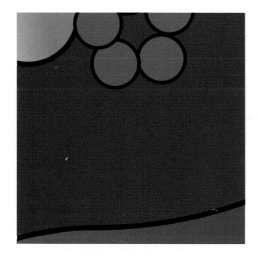

Minerals: Lending Strength and Glow to Good Health

THE SAME MINERALS that bolster metal buildings and the tallest mountains are crucial to human life. We know that our bodies need at least 24 minerals, and researchers are investigating roles additional minerals might play in good health. Some major minerals, calcium for example, are present in our bodies in amounts that weigh up to 2 or 3 pounds. The total of the trace minerals (those needed in very small quantities) is but a scant half-ounce, or the weight of three quarters.

Quantity doesn't enter into the equation tabulating the necessity of minerals, though. The 0.15 milligrams (far less than a billionth of an ounce) of iodine we need daily is no less critical to our health than the 1,000 to 1,500 milligrams of calcium essential to our bodies every day.

Minerals are required for such diverse functions as energy production, blood pressure regulation, heart muscle contraction, nerve conduction, wound healing, sperm formation, and labor in childbirth. In some cases, the combined effects of two or more minerals is more important than their singular actions. Conversely, one mineral may interfere with the absorption or function of another.

While minerals are decisively important to good health, getting more than the recommended amount can be dangerous. Arsenic, for example, is strategically important in small amounts but clearly poisonous at higher levels.

This chapter considers most minerals needed for good health, with two notable exceptions: calcium and iron. Because an increasing number of Americans' diets beg for more of these minerals, they're reserved for special consideration in Chapters 9 and 10.

Minerals are present in lots of different types of foods, and eating a varied, nutritious diet generally provides enough insurance against coming up short. In addition, most minerals are fairly indestructible, with few lost during storage and cooking.

Nutrition experts, however, warn that large numbers of Americans may be deficient in a growing cadre of minerals. Why? Two simple words explain the phenomenon: skimping and splurging. More and more people, especially women, are skimping on meat and dairy products in an attempt to cut down on dietary fat. Surveys reveal, in fact, that to reduce dietary fat many women cut out red meat and dairy products altogether (rather than choose lower-fat meats or fat-free dairy products). On the other hand, Americans are splurging on fast foods and other highly refined and processed foods—both shy on minerals—as they try to maximize shrinking free time.

According to nutrition surveys, about two-thirds of children and teens don't get enough *zinc*. In addition, the elderly, vegetarians, endurance athletes, diabetics, and alcoholics are at risk of becoming zinc deficient. This is cause for concern, since zinc is essential to many functions.

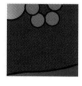

Beginning with its role in sperm production and the male sex hormone testosterone, zinc is of paramount importance in the formation of new life. It's also needed to replicate DNA, the genetic material that guides the formation and function of every living cell, critical of course to fetal growth (that's why zinc deficiency is particularly dangerous during pregnancy) as well as growth throughout infancy and childhood. In addition, zinc helps wounds heal, fights infection, and bolsters the immune system. Zinc is necessary to form healthy taste buds (which helps ensure a healthy appetite) and normal tissues lining the gastrointestinal tract. It's also vital in breaking down and using carbohydrates for fuel, as well as making proteins from the body's amino acid pool. Among its many other jobs, zinc is also fundamental to normal vision.

The best source of zinc is food of animal origin, such as meat and poultry (especially dark meat); other good sources include oysters, eggs, legumes, milk, and some whole-grain products. Including 2 cups milk, 5 servings of whole grains, 1 cup legumes, and 3 oz. of meat daily will supply your zinc requirement of 12 mg (or substitute an additional 1½ cups legumes for 3 oz. of meat). Because we hold very little zinc in storage, it's relatively easy to become zinc deficient.

Because *magnesium* is fundamental to so many key systems in the body, coming up short on magnesium can lead to serious health troubles. Although our bodies contain no more than one single ounce of magnesium, it's essential to keeping our hearts beating normally (deficiencies can lead to heart attack), muscles contracting, nerves functioning, and bones forming (working in concert with calcium and phosphorus). It's also indispensable in using and storing glucose, amino acids, and fatty acids, as well as in countless chemical, hormonal, and enzymatic reactions throughout the body. There's also some evidence that getting enough magnesium may prevent formation of some types of kidney stones. Vegetables, grains, milk, nuts, and legumes are all great sources of magnesium.

One of the greatest mineral success stories concerns *fluoride*. Since it was first added to drinking water in 1945, it has been credited with slashing the incidence of dental cavities by 40%. And now there's increasing evidence that when given in the correct mix with calcium, it can help restore bone in people with osteoporosis, a disease in which bones become brittle and break easily.

Unfortunately, though, fluoride has suffered from a bad reputation. Special interest groups opposed to water fluoridation have claimed that fluoride is responsible for cancer, mental retardation, and countless other conditions. But there's absolutely no evidence proving any of these claims. Too much fluoride can lead to discoloration of teeth and other problems, but such instances are rare.

The primary fluoride source for most people is fluoridated water. While it's seldom necessary to take a mineral supplement, a fluoride supplement may be in order if you live in an area without fluoridated water, especially for children. Check with your dentist.

Another mineral with widely divergent jobs, *phosphorus* is an integral ingredient of bone and teeth, as well as genetic material, cell membranes, and several enzymes. It's also indispensable in energy metabolism.

Because it's one of the only minerals readily abundant in processed foods (especially soft drinks and processed meats), there's growing concern that we may be getting *too much* phosphorus. While our bones demand an optimal ratio of 1 part phosphorus to 2 parts calcium, many diets contain far more phosphorus than calcium. This is especially true for a growing number of children, who consume soft drinks in place of milk. But eating a balanced diet containing meat, dairy products, grains, vegetables, and fruits should ensure the right ratio of dietary phosphorus to calcium.

Selenium, as a part of various enzymes, is another antioxidant warrior in the free-radical wars. In addition to helping fight off cancer, selenium helps the immune system and heart muscle function normally. Good sources of selenium include fish, meat, breads, and cereals.

Yet another mineral with widely diverse capabilities, *copper* helps make hemoglobin and collagen (supporting tissues throughout the body); maintains normal heart function and nerve transmission (because it's an ingredient of myelin, the protective sheath around nerve fibers); aids in blood clotting; regulates body temperature; strengthens bones; and, like many other minerals, is essential to glucose metabolism. There's also evidence that getting too little copper may contribute to mounting blood cholesterol levels. Copper may also bolster the immune system and thwart free-radical damage. Whole grains, liver, oysters, and nuts are good sources. Overdosing on vitamin C and zinc may interfere with copper absorption, so stay within recommended guidelines.

Chromium is intimately involved with energy metabolism, as well as regulating blood sugar levels—getting enough chromium may be especially important for individuals with diabetes. It is also essential in the transmission of genetic information and messages from one nerve cell to another. It may be important in reducing the effects of heart disease. Meats, cheese, brewer's yeast, dried beans, and whole grains are good sources of chromium.

Needed in extremely small amounts, *manganese* is another key ingredient in bone formation; it's also essential to the nervous system, normal reproduction, and protein and energy metabolism. As with other minerals, stay within recommended guidelines, as too much can interfere with iron absorption. Whole grains, legumes, and liver are rich in manganese.

There's also definitive evidence that we need sulfur, chlorine, potassium, sodium, and molybdenum, and mounting evidence we need boron, nickel, vanadium, arsenic, cobalt, lithium, silicon, tin, and cadmium.

A note on supplements: As with other nutrients, strive to get your minerals from food. Fashioning an eating plan of lots of fruits, vegetables, whole grains, and some dairy foods and some meat will deliver all the minerals you need. Not only are the extra in supplements useless, but they may be harmful.

How the Body Gets Minerals

Minerals are found freely in nature and eventually wind their way into our food supply, some accumulating in certain foods, and others in other types of food. Here's how and where to find them.

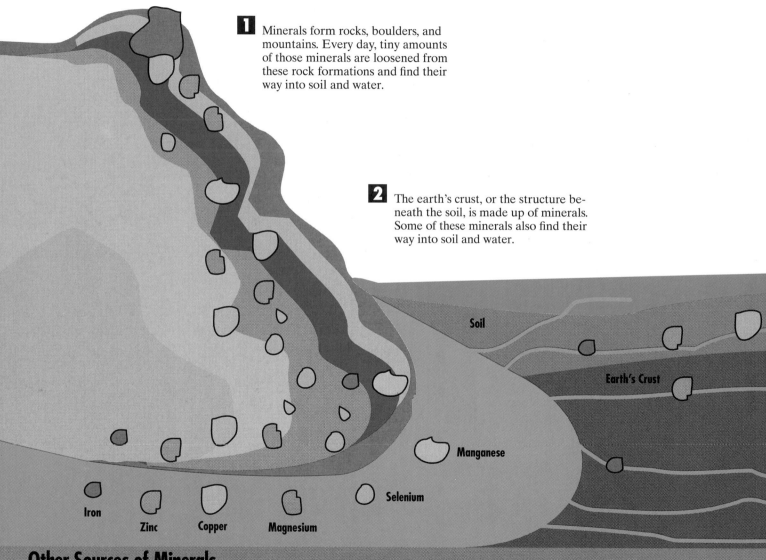

1 Minerals form rocks, boulders, and mountains. Every day, tiny amounts of those minerals are loosened from these rock formations and find their way into soil and water.

2 The earth's crust, or the structure beneath the soil, is made up of minerals. Some of these minerals also find their way into soil and water.

Soil

Earth's Crust

Manganese

Selenium

Iron

Zinc

Copper

Magnesium

Other Sources of Minerals

Legumes This complex carbohydrate package shines again, boasting a good mineral content. Legumes, such as lentils and split peas, are great sources of zinc, magnesium, manganese, and molybdenum.

Fluoridated Water This is the best source of fluoride, the mineral credited with slashing the incidence of dental cavities by 40%. If your water isn't fluoridated, or your children drink mostly bottled water, ask your dentist about a supplement.

Nuts Sprinkle a few nuts into your diet to help you harvest enough magnesium and copper. Remember, though, nuts are high in fat!

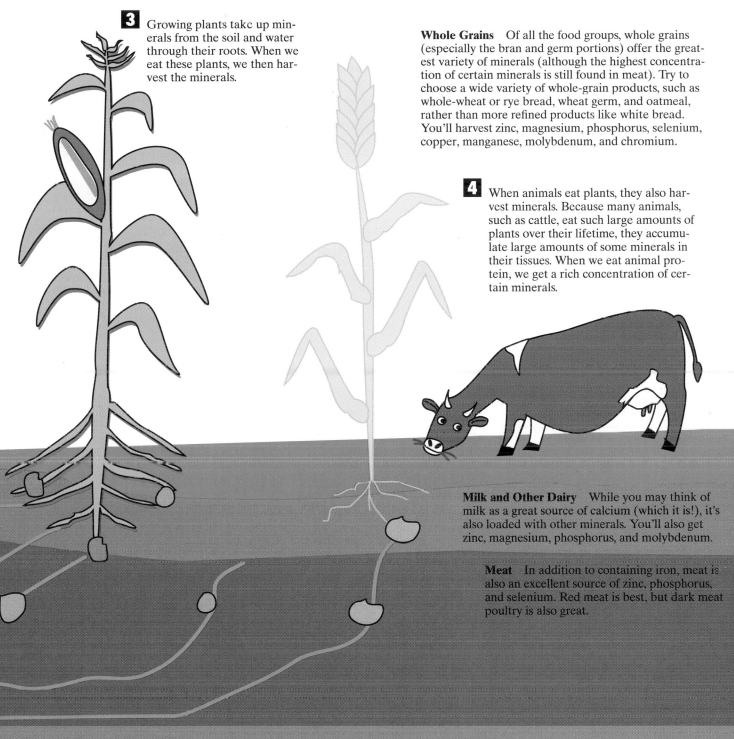

3 Growing plants take up minerals from the soil and water through their roots. When we eat these plants, we then harvest the minerals.

Whole Grains   Of all the food groups, whole grains (especially the bran and germ portions) offer the greatest variety of minerals (although the highest concentration of certain minerals is still found in meat). Try to choose a wide variety of whole-grain products, such as whole-wheat or rye bread, wheat germ, and oatmeal, rather than more refined products like white bread. You'll harvest zinc, magnesium, phosphorus, selenium, copper, manganese, molybdenum, and chromium.

4 When animals eat plants, they also harvest minerals. Because many animals, such as cattle, eat such large amounts of plants over their lifetime, they accumulate large amounts of some minerals in their tissues. When we eat animal protein, we get a rich concentration of certain minerals.

Milk and Other Dairy   While you may think of milk as a great source of calcium (which it is!), it's also loaded with other minerals. You'll also get zinc, magnesium, phosphorus, and molybdenum.

Meat   In addition to containing iron, meat is also an excellent source of zinc, phosphorus, and selenium. Red meat is best, but dark meat poultry is also great.

Fish   Catching a fish meal now and then will boost selenium intake. Oysters are loaded with zinc and copper.

Iodized Salt   Be sure to use iodized salt (although not to excess—see Chapter 14) to make sure you're getting enough iodine.

Try a New Food   Some unusual foods are fabulous sources of several minerals. Cassava, tamarinds, and watercress are loaded with calcium, phosphorus, magnesium, and potassium. Check them out!

Minerals Everywhere! For Example, How the Body Uses Copper

Minerals are at work in every cell throughout the body, serving as important ingredients of many cells and tissues and critical regulators of many body processes. Minerals take on such diverse roles as forming bone tissue and making sure nerve cells transmit the messages that control our thoughts and movements. Here, we look at one example, copper, and just some of its many and varied jobs in the human body. (In addition to what's pictured here, copper has many other responsibilities, including preventing damage by free radicals and aiding in iron absorption.)

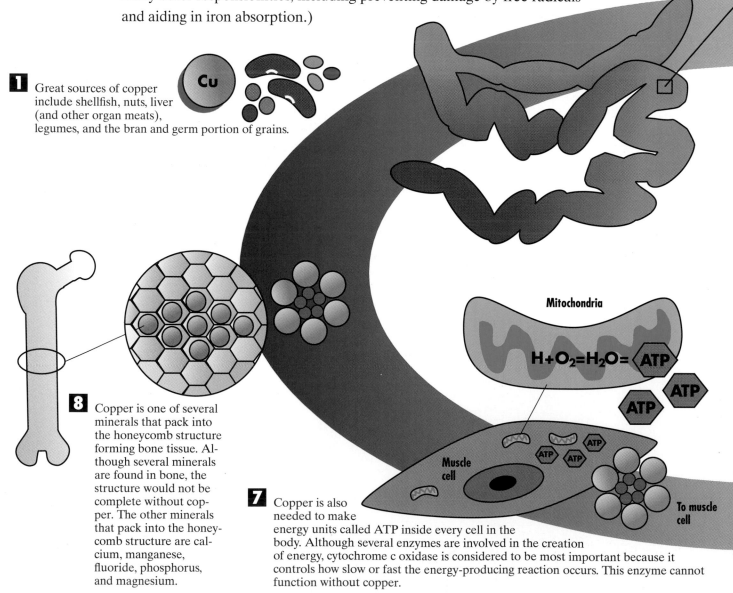

1 Great sources of copper include shellfish, nuts, liver (and other organ meats), legumes, and the bran and germ portion of grains.

Cu

Mitochondria

$H+O_2=H_2O=$ ATP

ATP

ATP

ATP

ATP

ATP ATP

Muscle cell

To muscle cell

8 Copper is one of several minerals that pack into the honeycomb structure forming bone tissue. Although several minerals are found in bone, the structure would not be complete without copper. The other minerals that pack into the honeycomb structure are calcium, manganese, fluoride, phosphorus, and magnesium.

7 Copper is also needed to make energy units called ATP inside every cell in the body. Although several enzymes are involved in the creation of energy, cytochrome c oxidase is considered to be most important because it controls how slow or fast the energy-producing reaction occurs. This enzyme cannot function without copper.

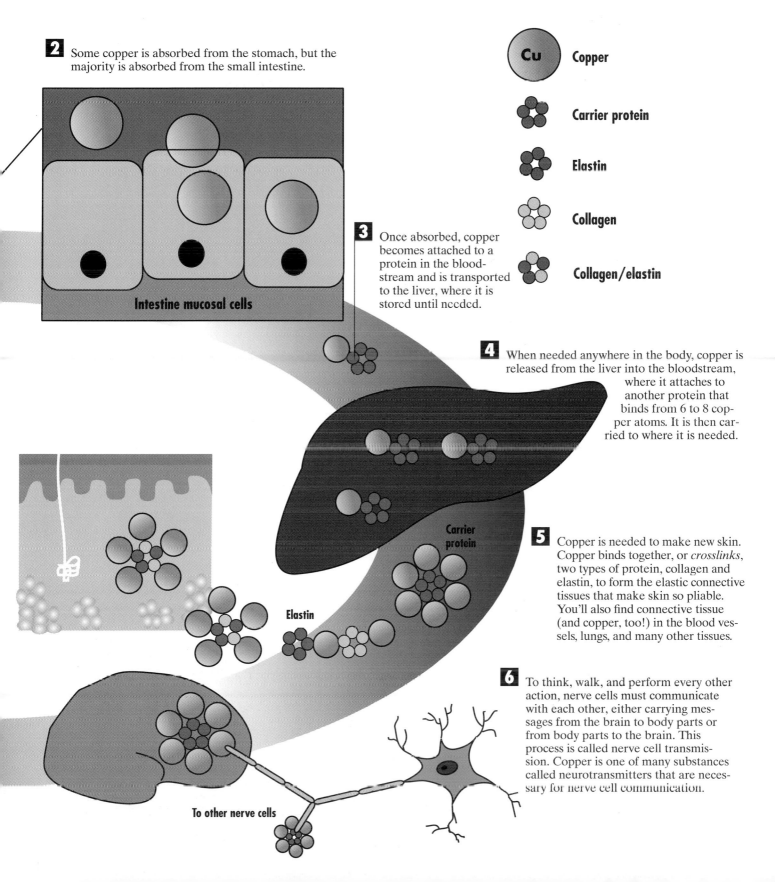

2 Some copper is absorbed from the stomach, but the majority is absorbed from the small intestine.

Intestine mucosal cells

Cu **Copper**

Carrier protein

Elastin

Collagen

Collagen/elastin

3 Once absorbed, copper becomes attached to a protein in the bloodstream and is transported to the liver, where it is stored until needed.

4 When needed anywhere in the body, copper is released from the liver into the bloodstream, where it attaches to another protein that binds from 6 to 8 copper atoms. It is then carried to where it is needed.

Carrier protein

Elastin

5 Copper is needed to make new skin. Copper binds together, or *crosslinks*, two types of protein, collagen and elastin, to form the elastic connective tissues that make skin so pliable. You'll also find connective tissue (and copper, too!) in the blood vessels, lungs, and many other tissues.

6 To think, walk, and perform every other action, nerve cells must communicate with each other, either carrying messages from the brain to body parts or from body parts to the brain. This process is called nerve cell transmission. Copper is one of many substances called neurotransmitters that are necessary for nerve cell communication.

To other nerve cells

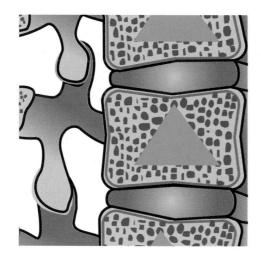

CHAPTER

9

Calcium: More Than Strong Bones

WHETHER YOU'RE 8, 28, or 88, the amount of calcium in your diet affects the strength of your bones, now and in the future.

In this country, there's a virtual epidemic of weak bones, or osteoporosis, which forever changes its victim's lifestyle and physical abilities. Women are the primary victims—as many as half of American women over age 45 have osteoporosis. Osteoporosis can even lead to death—as many as 20% of all people who suffer a hip fracture, one consequence of osteoporosis, die within a year from associated complications.

While many minerals and some vitamins contribute to bone strength, calcium is the quintessential mineral dictating strength—it's the single most important nutritional influence on how dense bones become (gender, race, and genetics are unchangeable influences). But calcium is also needed for several other vital functions, including muscle contraction, blood clotting, and immune competence—the body's self-defense mechanism against infection; it also plays a variety of regulatory roles in every living cell. Although just 1% of the body's calcium is found outside of bone, it is these other functions that take precedence over calcium's role in building and maintaining bone strength. That fact takes on critical importance: When we don't take in enough calcium, the body draws calcium from bone to fulfill these other vital functions. Over time, this can lead to weaker bones. Calcium loss is accelerated by two other factors: aging and menopause.

Here's a more intimate look at calcium's role in bone health, and how aging and menopause figure in. Like the steel framework that reinforces a skyscraper, your skeleton serves as the body's framework. If the framework is not strong enough, the entire building can crack and crumble. If bones become osteoporotic, or fragile, they'll break very easily—sneezing may be enough to fracture vertebrae, or backbones.

However, unlike the lifeless metal that reinforces that skyscraper, the human skeleton is a constantly changing, living tissue—a honeycomb-type structure packed full of calcium and mineral deposits. From the day we are born to the day we die, our bones undergo a process called remodeling—breaking down old bone and replacing it with strong new bone.

Early in life, bone replacement exceeds bone breakdown as calcium and other minerals are added to the honeycomb structure. That's why bones continue to grow in length and density through our teen years. After that, the density continues to increase well into our third decade of life. That's right: Contrary to what many people believe, bones still need calcium to grow stronger after they finish growing in length. Bones require extra calcium until sometime into our 30s, when they are as dense and as strong as they'll ever be, or they've reached peak bone mass.

This is a critical point. How dense a person's bones are when peak bone mass is reached determines a person's risk of fracture later in life. There's no doubt that people with higher peak bone mass have far fewer fractures later in life compared to people with lower peak bone masses. Why?

Sometime around age 40, the process reverses and calcium and other minerals begin to leave that honeycomb structure faster than new ones can take their place. Just as a matter of aging, our bones can lose around one-half to one percent of their mass per year—unless we do something about it.

On top of that, women are hit with an even more dramatic bone loss after menopause when estrogen levels decline. That's because estrogen helps the bones "hang on" to calcium. In just the 3 to 5 years following the onset of menopause, a woman can lose up to 15% of bone mass. Coupled with the bone loss of aging, a woman can lose up to a quarter or even half of her peak bone mass by age 80. Women with denser bones, however, stand a better chance of remaining strong even after these bone-robbing assaults. And although estrogen-related bone loss cannot be stopped, the bone loss of aging *can*.

In what's been called one of the greatest medical advances of the decade, there's now sufficient evidence that getting enough calcium after age 40—right through to the last years of life—will stop the gradual chipping away of bone that is otherwise a normal part of aging. This is even true for postmenopausal women!

How much calcium is enough? More than nutrition experts previously thought. Although the U.S. RDA for calcium is 1,200 milligrams up to the age of 24 and 800 after age 24, leading calcium experts recommend that premenopausal women over age 30 and men of all ages should aim for 1,000 milligrams daily and postmenopausal women should consume no less than 1,500 milligrams daily. In sharp contrast, most women aged 20 to 50 consume an average of 600 milligrams daily, and postmenopausal women just 500 milligrams.

In studies, postmenopausal women who got a least 1,500 milligrams of calcium daily lost just one-third to one-half as much bone as women who didn't get enough calcium. Experts say this cumulative "bone savings" quickly makes a big difference. In just 18 months, women getting at least 1,500 milligrams of calcium daily will have notably fewer fractures than women getting 750 milligrams or less.

As with every other nutrient, the best source of calcium is food. Milk and other dairy products are the best source, and some vegetables have small amounts of calcium the body can absorb. They include broccoli, kale, cabbage, watercress, and radishes. Other vegetables, such as spinach, rhubarb, chard, and beet greens have moderate amounts of calcium, but also contain oxalic acid, a substance that binds calcium, rendering it unabsorbable.

But getting enough calcium from food may be difficult, especially for women who limit calories. One cup of milk or yogurt, for example, has 300 milligrams, ½ cup of the vegetables mentioned above has 10–50 milligrams; an ounce of cheese has 100–200 milligrams; and 6 ounces of calcium-fortified orange juice has around 200 milligrams. If you cannot get enough calcium from food, especially if you're a woman, be sure to take a calcium supplement. Although nutrient supplements are very seldom warranted, this is one case in which they can virtually change a person's life.

If you're turning to a calcium supplement, you may instinctively reach for natural sources like dolomite, bonemeal, or crushed oyster shells. But these sources may be dangerously laden with lead and other toxic minerals. Reach instead for a laboratory-produced version. Calcium carbonate may be your best bet, as it is the most concentrated source of calcium. Take your supplement with food to increase absorption.

In addition to getting enough calcium, be sure to get enough vitamin D, which helps absorb calcium, and avoid an excessively fatty diet, alcohol, and tobacco, all of which tend to promote calcium loss. Excessively high protein or salt intake also robs bones of calcium, so stick to healthy-size doses of each. While the equivalent of 2 or 3 cups of caffeine-containing coffee a day doesn't seem to promote calcium loss, excessive caffeine intake can. If you're a woman, check with your doctor about estrogen replacement therapy after menopause; this works extremely well to conserve calcium. Finally, you can hang on to the calcium (and other minerals) in your bones by exercising with the weight of gravity (walking is exercising with the weight of gravity, swimming is not).

Beyond warding off osteoporosis and supporting vital chemical reactions, calcium helps keep blood pressure at a healthy low reading, and there's mounting evidence that it fights off colon cancer. New evidence is emerging that calcium may offer two other benefits: It may help ease the physical and emotional discomforts that trouble some women premenstrually; and one study of men on high-calcium diets found calcium had a cholesterol-lowering effect.

How the Body Uses Calcium

Calcium deficiency creates one of the most serious public health problems: osteoporosis. Women, who are especially prone to developing osteoporosis, can ensure that they'll have a healthy, active life in their later years by getting enough calcium throughout their lives. Here's how calcium works in the body.

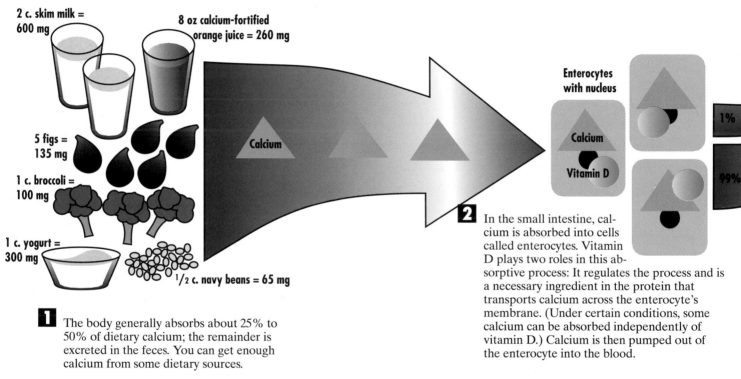

2 c. skim milk = 600 mg

8 oz calcium-fortified orange juice = 260 mg

5 figs = 135 mg

1 c. broccoli = 100 mg

1 c. yogurt = 300 mg

1/2 c. navy beans = 65 mg

Calcium

Enterocytes with nucleus

Calcium

Vitamin D

1%

99%

1 The body generally absorbs about 25% to 50% of dietary calcium; the remainder is excreted in the feces. You can get enough calcium from some dietary sources.

2 In the small intestine, calcium is absorbed into cells called enterocytes. Vitamin D plays two roles in this absorptive process: It regulates the process and is a necessary ingredient in the protein that transports calcium across the enterocyte's membrane. (Under certain conditions, some calcium can be absorbed independently of vitamin D.) Calcium is then pumped out of the enterocyte into the blood.

11 Menopause induces another type of bone loss. When a woman's estrogen levels drop after menopause, she begins to lose bone mass, especially in the backbones, or vertebrae. This is why postmenopausal women are so prone to breaking their vertebrae by such simple actions as sneezing or lifting a basket of laundry. These are often called compression fractures; with each such fracture, height is lost. Gradual loss of bone density and an increasing number of spinal compression fractures lead to a loss of height over the years.

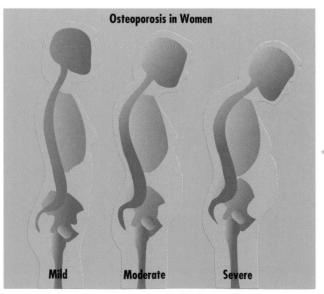

Osteoporosis in Women

Mild   **Moderate**   **Severe**

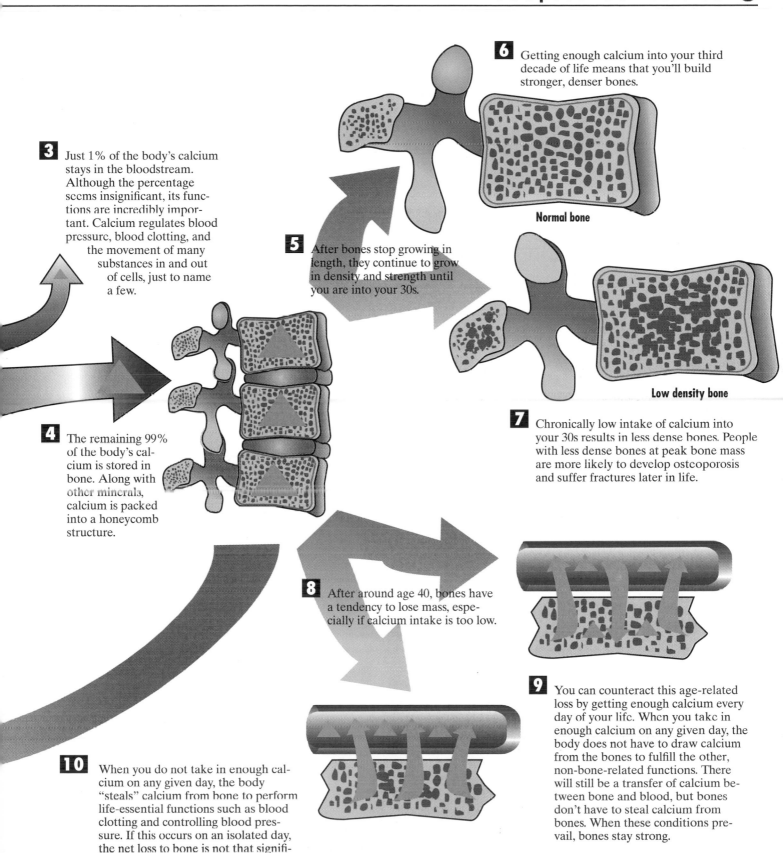

3 Just 1% of the body's calcium stays in the bloodstream. Although the percentage seems insignificant, its functions are incredibly important. Calcium regulates blood pressure, blood clotting, and the movement of many substances in and out of cells, just to name a few.

4 The remaining 99% of the body's calcium is stored in bone. Along with other minerals, calcium is packed into a honeycomb structure.

5 After bones stop growing in length, they continue to grow in density and strength until you are into your 30s.

6 Getting enough calcium into your third decade of life means that you'll build stronger, denser bones.

Normal bone

Low density bone

7 Chronically low intake of calcium into your 30s results in less dense bones. People with less dense bones at peak bone mass are more likely to develop osteoporosis and suffer fractures later in life.

8 After around age 40, bones have a tendency to lose mass, especially if calcium intake is too low.

9 You can counteract this age-related loss by getting enough calcium every day of your life. When you take in enough calcium on any given day, the body does not have to draw calcium from the bones to fulfill the other, non-bone-related functions. There will still be a transfer of calcium between bone and blood, but bones don't have to steal calcium from bones. When these conditions prevail, bones stay strong.

10 When you do not take in enough calcium on any given day, the body "steals" calcium from bone to perform life-essential functions such as blood clotting and controlling blood pressure. If this occurs on an isolated day, the net loss to bone is not that significant. But chronic loss leads to weakened, or osteoporotic bones.

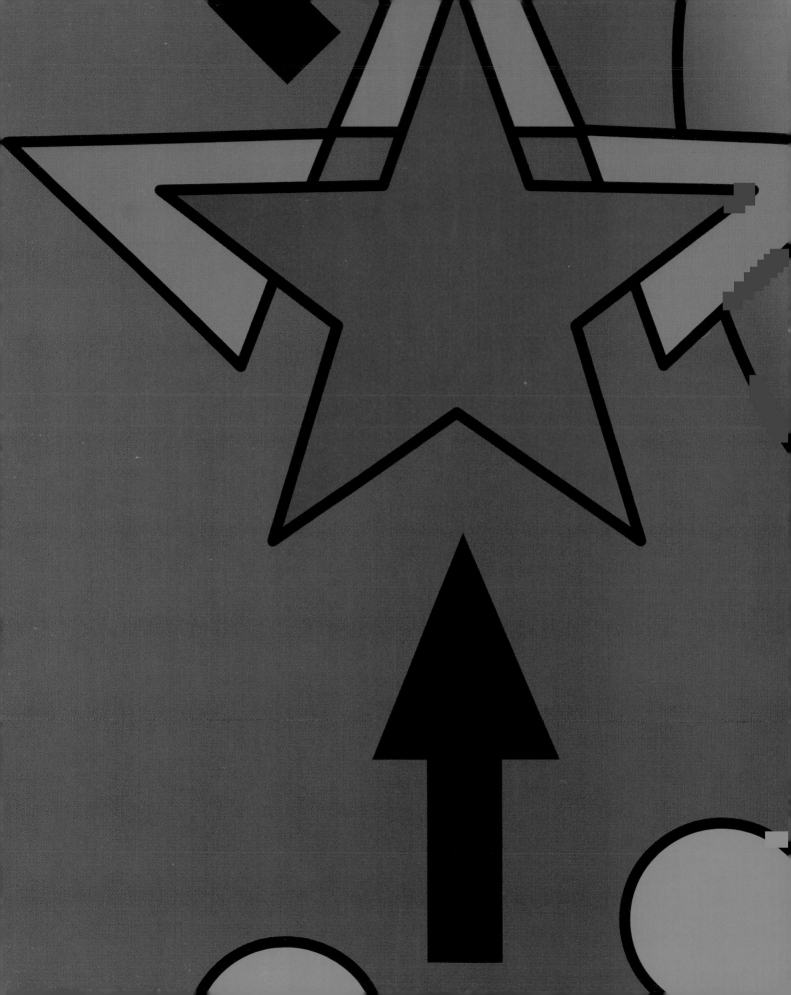

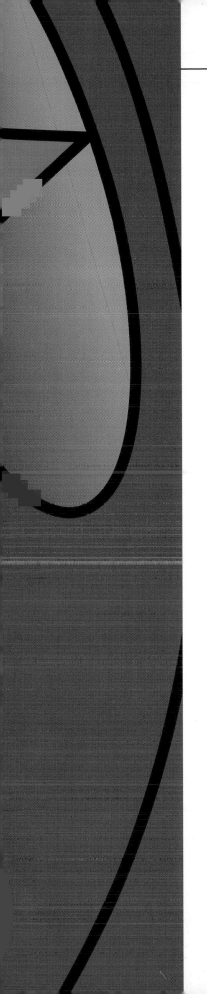

HOW TO WIN YOUR NUTRITION BATTLES

CONTENTS

Chapter 10   Iron: How to Prevent the Most Common
Nutritional Deficiency
90

Chapter 11   Nutrient Density: More Nutrition per Calorie
98

Chapter 12   Fat: Both Friend and Foe
104

Chapter 13   How to Eat to Lower Cholesterol: Fact and Fad
112

Chapter 14   Re-salt Your Diet to Control Blood Pressure
124

Chapter 15   How to Get Enough Fiber to Fight Disease
132

Chapter 16   How to Stop Dieting and Be Trim
140

Chapter 17   How to Fight Cancer with a Healthy Diet
146

Chapter 18   You Still Have Questions
154

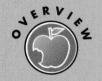

OVERVIEW

T'S ONE THING to know about good nutrition and quite another to put the knowledge into practice every day. We sometimes feel as though we have forever to institute the sound nutrition practices presented in this book—as we run through the fast-food drive-up window for a third time in a week, or skip a vegetable at dinner *again*. Of course we all want to achieve optimal health and energy, but when you're motivated by a more specific reason, the desire to practice good nutrition becomes especially compelling.

For example, people with a family history of heart disease may want to know if they can eat so as to minimize their own risk of developing heart disease. Someone with hypertension wants to know how to modify diet to lower blood pressure—and reduce risk for stroke and heart attack. Most people want to know how to eat to minimize cancer risk. Last, and certainly not least, those engaged in the battle of the bulge want to know how to end the battle and win the war.

As you read the following chapters, remember that you can win 99% of your nutrition battles with good food—without using any "health foods" or supplements. Also note that you can't solve any nutrition battle in a vacuum, that each nutrition problem or battle is related to every other. If, for example, you drink an excessive quantity of soda pop, you may have a problem with your weight from all the extra calories. You'll most likely also have a problem with your calcium intake (placing you at risk for osteoporosis, or brittle bones) because you're probably drinking pop to the exclusion of calcium rich milk. You may also come up critically short on other nutrients if you bypass fruits and vegetables for soda pop.

Similarly, if you're dousing your food with olive oil because you've heard that it protects against heart disease, you'll no doubt develop a weight problem from all the extra calories, and you'll probably also have an *elevated* blood cholesterol.

Read on to see how to win *your* nutrition battles.

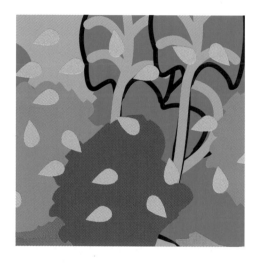

CHAPTER 10

Iron: How to Prevent the Most Common Nutritional Deficiency

N EVERY CORNER of the world, more people suffer from iron deficiency than from any other nutrient deficiency. Some 35–55% of young, healthy women are iron deficient; the incidence is even higher among pregnant women who do not take iron. In addition, 6–12% of children aged 1–14 years are iron deficient. While the majority of iron-deficient people don't suffer severe symptoms—shortness of breath, weakness, and paleness—most suffer the subtler signs of fatigue, headaches, and irritability.

Iron's most important job is forming red blood cells. Nearly three-quarters of the iron in our body, in fact, is found in a segment of the red blood cells called hemoglobin. Hemoglobin carries oxygen from the lungs to every tissue and cell in the body, which need the oxygen to drive energy-producing reactions, as well as many other chemical reactions that keep the body functioning normally. For example, iron is a key player in energy-regulating enzymes; it plays a role in building a strong immune system that can fight infections; it helps convert beta carotene into vitamin A; it's necessary to remove fats from blood; and, last but not least, iron helps the liver detoxify chemical substances.

Getting enough iron is not as easy as counting up the milligrams of iron in the food you eat. That's because iron absorption is complicated by several factors, which means the body only absorbs a portion of dietary iron. Here's what affects iron absorption.

The type of iron in a particular food. Meat and fish contain heme iron, a form of iron that is more readily absorbed than nonheme iron (found in grains, fruits, vegetables, and dairy foods). Overall, just 2% to 20% of nonheme iron is absorbed, compared to 10% to 35% of heme iron.

Iron inhibitors. Many foods containing nonheme iron have naturally occurring substances (collectively called ligands) that bind up the iron, making it unavailable for absorption (heme iron isn't affected by these ligands). In addition, some foods with sources of nonheme iron can bind up the nonheme iron of another food when eaten in the same meal. Wheat and rice, for example, contain ligands that bind up most of the nonheme iron found in kidney beans. Other foods known for binding up iron include coffee, tea (reduces nonheme iron absorption by as much as 60%), spinach, legumes, and chocolate. Of particular interest to women, calcium also inhibits iron absorption. Experts recommend that people take calcium supplements at a time other than when they are eating iron-rich foods or taking an iron supplement.

Iron enhancers. Meat contains substances that enhance absorption of nonheme iron. Eating a little meat, fish, or poultry with nonheme sources of iron increases the absorption of nonheme iron as much as two to four times. In addition to meat, other substances increase nonheme iron absorption: namely, citric acid, lactic acid, and—most especially—ascorbic acid or vitamin C. Foods high in ascorbic acid, such as orange juice can increase the absorption of nonheme iron by as much as 85% when consumed at the same time.

How much iron the body needs. Iron-deficient people absorb more iron—sometimes over twice as much—than do those with iron-rich blood.

Even people who eat a healthy, balanced diet are at higher risk of iron deficiency during certain times of the life cycle. Infants and children are at risk because of rapid growth; children aged 9 to 18 months are especially prone to developing iron-deficiency anemia because of the growth spurt they undergo at this time. Iron-deficiency anemia is also common during the adolescent growth spurt (especially among menstruating girls). In some children, a poor diet, such as one containing too much milk, also contributes to the development of iron deficiency. (When children drink too much milk, they simply don't have room for other foods that do have iron.)

Menstruating women lose significant amounts of iron every month, and women who bleed heavily have an especially hard time getting enough iron from diet alone. Pregnant women have significantly higher iron requirements to support their own needs as well as those of their growing baby. Dieters, especially chronic dieters, simply don't take in enough calories to get enough iron. Strict vegetarians are at risk because many don't take in enough iron, and even those who do may not be able to absorb the iron because of the ligands, or substances that inhibit iron absorption, discussed above. Some experts recommend that strict vegetarians who rely on vegetarian sources of iron exclusively consume more iron than meat eaters.

These high-risk groups should pay special attention to getting enough iron and should even consider an iron supplement.

Iron deficiency, especially in children, is dangerous for many reasons beyond the obvious. In addition to suffering more infections, gastrointestinal abnormalities, and weakened muscles, iron-deficient children have a greatly impaired ability to learn and suffer more behavior problems. Alarmingly, these learning deficits can occur even with relatively mild iron-deficiency anemia, and researchers are uncertain about their reversibility. Although the exact mechanism by which this occurs is not known, it is believed that a lack of iron causes defects in chemicals involved in neural transmission, or nerve cell communication.

Although research is not conclusive, some studies have shown that these iron-deficiency–associated cognitive difficulties may even occur in adults. One study showed that iron-deficient adults were viewed by their supervisors as lazy and unintelligent, but after receiving iron supplements they came to be viewed as bright, motivated, and productive.

To get more iron and to make the most of the iron you do eat, try to do the following: Eat a little meat, fish, or poultry five times per week (where each serving is 3–4 ounces). When eating vegetable sources of iron, also eat a food high in ascorbic acid, such as citrus fruits, or try to include just a little meat. For example, even just a token amount of ground beef in chili enhances absorption of iron from kidney beans. If you depend totally on vegetable sources of iron, try to include a good source at each meal, and also aim for a little more than the RDA. Do not take calcium supplements with a meal high in iron. Try to cook acidic foods, such as any tomato-based recipe (spaghetti sauce, chili, and so on) in an iron pan. Some of the iron will leach into the food; the longer food simmers, the more iron will be leached.

How to Get a Day's Worth of Iron—and Absorb More of It

Getting enough iron is difficult, especially for menstruating women. Make a point of eating iron-rich foods *and* eating nonmeat sources of iron with foods that help increase absorption, such as acidic foods like orange juice and tomatoes. Here's one way a menstruating woman can get a day's worth of iron and absorb more of it.

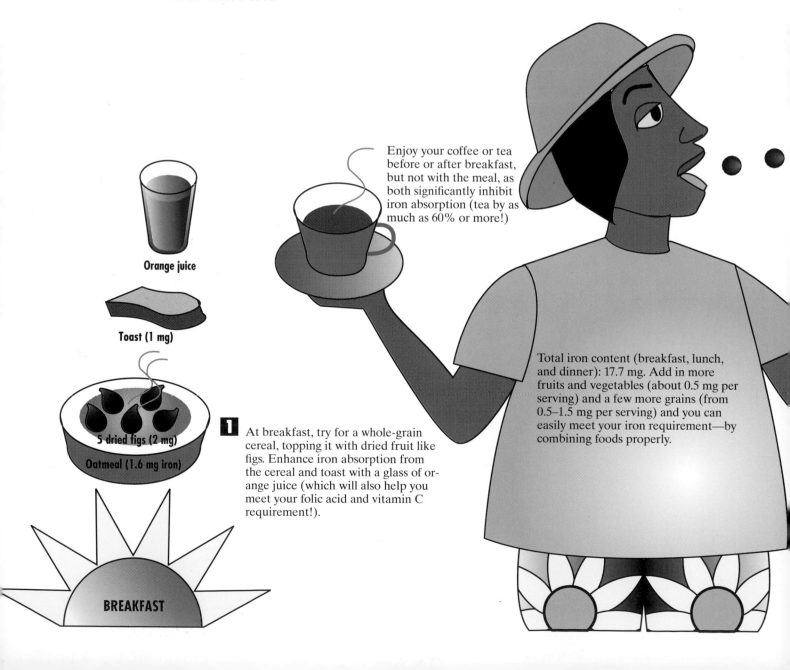

Orange juice

Toast (1 mg)

5 dried figs (2 mg)

Oatmeal (1.6 mg iron)

Enjoy your coffee or tea before or after breakfast, but not with the meal, as both significantly inhibit iron absorption (tea by as much as 60% or more!)

1 At breakfast, try for a whole-grain cereal, topping it with dried fruit like figs. Enhance iron absorption from the cereal and toast with a glass of orange juice (which will also help you meet your folic acid and vitamin C requirement!).

Total iron content (breakfast, lunch, and dinner): 17.7 mg. Add in more fruits and vegetables (about 0.5 mg per serving) and a few more grains (from 0.5–1.5 mg per serving) and you can easily meet your iron requirement—by combining foods properly.

BREAKFAST

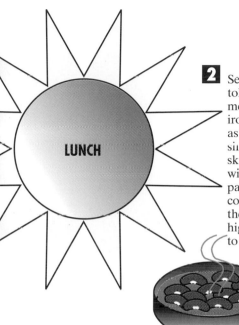

2 Serving up chili for lunch? Add in a token dash of lean ground beef, as meat helps you absorb the nonheme iron in vegetable sources of iron such as the kidney beans in chili. Also, simmer chili all morning in an iron skillet, as the acid from the tomatoes will leach some of the iron from the pan into the food, boosting the iron content of your chili. Just to be on the safe side, finish your meal with a high–vitamin C fruit like cantaloupe to further bolster iron absorption.

Chili
1 c. kidney beans (3.3 mg)
1 oz. hamburger (.8 mg)

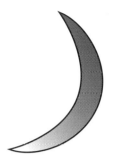

Sweet potato (.5 mg)

Salad with 1 oz. sesame seeds (4 mg)

4 Need to take a calcium supplement? (Most women do!) Don't take it with meals high in iron, as each mineral interferes with the absorption of the other. When should you take your calcium? Try between meals, with a little orange juice or something else acidic to help you absorb it.

Corn bread (1 mg)

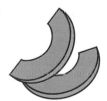

1 c. cantaloupe (.3 mg)

3 Try to include a little meat—3 to 4 ounces—at least five times per week. Red meat has more iron than does poultry or fish, but the iron in all of these flesh foods is readily absorbed and not affected by dietary substances that inhibit nonheme sources of iron (iron in vegetable foods).

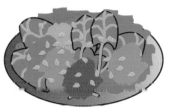

1 c. pearl barley (2 mg)

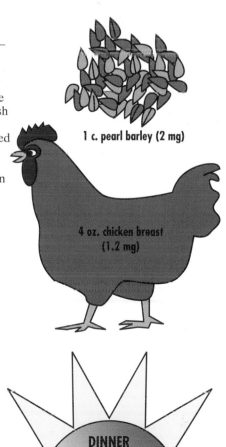

4 oz. chicken breast (1.2 mg)

DINNER

How Much Iron Do I Need?

Infants (full-term)	0–3 months	—*
	3–6 months	6.6 mg
	6–12 months	8.8 mg
Children	1–10 years	10 mg
Males	10–18 years	12 mg
	18+	10 mg
Females	Non-pregnant 10–45 years	15 mg
	Pregnant	30 mg
	Post-menopausal	10 mg

* Infants store enough before birth to last about 3 months.

How the Body Uses and Reuses Iron

Every body needs enough iron for many critical functions. Prime among them are carrying oxygen from the lungs to cells to make energy, and carrying the potentially dangerous carbon dioxide waste product away from cells to be excreted through the lungs. Iron-deficient people—even those who are not anemic—experience subtle symptoms of fatigue and irritability that can interfere with their ability to learn and work efficiently. Here's what the body does with iron, and how it recycles it over and over again.

2 Between two-thirds and three-fourths of the body's iron is found in hemoglobin, a component of red blood cells. When the body needs to make red blood cells, iron is transported to the bone marrow, where red blood cells are formed. (During iron deficiency, the body makes more transferrin so as to be able to transport more iron to marrow.) Excess iron is carried to the liver, spleen, or bone marrow, where it is stored for later use.

Hip bone

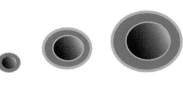

Iron

Intestine epithelial cells

Transferrin

1 Iron is absorbed by epithelial cells in the small intestine. The iron is transferred into the blood, where it hooks up with a protein called transferrin, whose job is to transport the iron around the body to where it's needed.

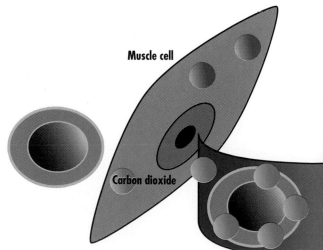

Muscle cell

Carbon dioxide

8 The red blood cell continues to work this way for approximately four months, its normal life span. Then, the worn-out red blood cell is destroyed and the iron is released to begin the cycle over again. In men and nonmenstruating women, iron losses are much smaller than in menstruating women. Other conditions that cause blood loss, such as disease or injury, increase iron loss and therefore increase iron needs.

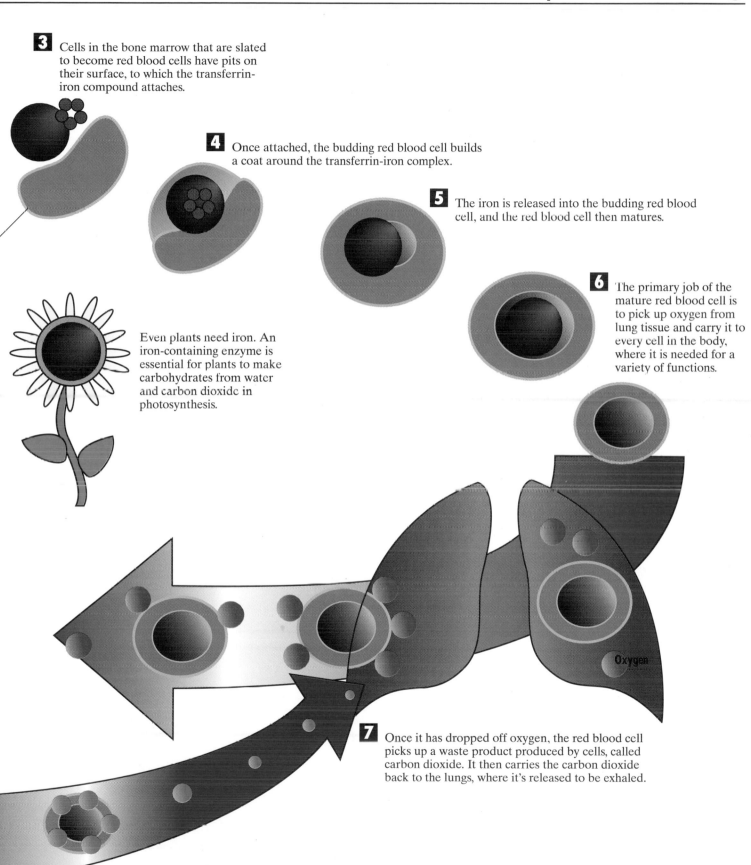

3 Cells in the bone marrow that are slated to become red blood cells have pits on their surface, to which the transferrin-iron compound attaches.

4 Once attached, the budding red blood cell builds a coat around the transferrin-iron complex.

5 The iron is released into the budding red blood cell, and the red blood cell then matures.

6 The primary job of the mature red blood cell is to pick up oxygen from lung tissue and carry it to every cell in the body, where it is needed for a variety of functions.

Even plants need iron. An iron-containing enzyme is essential for plants to make carbohydrates from water and carbon dioxide in photosynthesis.

Oxygen

7 Once it has dropped off oxygen, the red blood cell picks up a waste product produced by cells, called carbon dioxide. It then carries the carbon dioxide back to the lungs, where it's released to be exhaled.

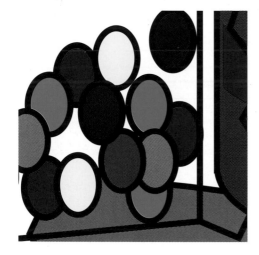

CHAPTER 11

Nutrient Density: More Nutrition per Calorie

WHEN YOU GO to the grocery store, do you try to get the most for your money? Do you shop carefully, comparing prices so that you'll pack your grocery bags with the most food per dollar spent? You should also compare foods for their nutrient content, trying to select the best nutrition "buys." In other words, you should be concerned about *nutrient density.* And then you'll be able to spend your calories as wisely as you do your money.

Foods that are nutritionally dense are rich in vitamins and minerals—they have more nutrients per calorie than do other foods. Nutritionally dense foods stand in stark contrast to empty-calorie foods, which are generally loaded with fat and refined sugar and stripped of most vitamins and minerals. Soda pop, most candy, potato chips, and many other snack foods are empty-calorie foods. Empty-calorie foods use up your calorie allowance quickly, with almost no nutritional payoff.

Here are some examples of nutritionally dense foods, compared to their less dense counterparts. A baked potato is more nutritionally dense than potato chips. Romaine lettuce is a powerhouse of nutrition compared with pale iceberg. And some foods have good amounts of nutrients, but they're diluted in lots of extra calories, making them less nutritionally dense foods. Three ounces of fried chicken, for example, is far less nutritionally dense than 3 ounces of roasted chicken. You can get 26 grams of protein, 80% of your niacin RDA, 30% of your selenium RDA, and 30% of your B-6 RDA for just 139 calories of skinless, roasted chicken breast, compared with 220 calories if you leave the skin on and fry that chicken breast. One cup of whole milk is less nutritionally dense than one cup of skim milk. Ditto for one cup of nonfat yogurt with syrupy fruit compared with one cup of nonfat yogurt topped with sliced fresh fruit. When it comes to fruits and vegetables, generally the richly colored foods are more nutritionally dense than their paler counterparts.

While everyone should be concerned about nutrient density, certain groups of people should be especially tuned in to selecting nutritionally dense foods, the elderly prime among them. As we age, we need fewer and fewer calories (because every year beginning around age 40 we lose active muscle tissue, which means we need a decreasing number of calories) but just as many nutrients. The elderly, in fact, are frequently deficient in one or more nutrients, simply because they eat less food and far fewer nutrients. Similarly, people who are trying to lose weight focus in on lowering the calorie content of their diet, often with little concern for nutrients (how many dieters do you know who reserve 200–300 calories for a special gooey dessert?)—which means they also simultaneously slash their nutrient intake.

But it *is* possible to cut down on excess calories and still get the nutrition you need—simply by choosing more nutritionally dense foods. To achieve or maintain a healthy body weight, try eating with nutrient density in mind. It's a wonderful alternative to counting calories.

Choosing a nutritionally dense food over a nutritionally weak one is just the first way of taking nutrient density into account. The second way is to avoid diluting nutritionally dense foods. For example, using too much salad dressing with nutritionally dense foods like romaine lettuce and kidney beans lessens your nutrient density for that day. As another example, instead of topping your whole-wheat toast with margarine and jelly, cover it with nonfat ricotta cheese and fresh strawberry slices; you'll have eaten fewer calories while bolstering your protein, vitamin C, and fiber intake. Not diluting nutritionally dense foods by adding in empty calories gives you a better nutrition picture.

And now for the third consideration: Try for nutrient variety as well as density. A preposterous example illustrates the point. Eating 15 bananas in one day definitely yields a greater nutrient density than drinking 15 cans of soda pop (calories are approximately equal in each case). But you'll have a tremendously high intake of certain nutrients, and nearly none of others.

To ensure density in nutrient variety, choose at least 10 to 15 different foods each day, handpicking the nutritionally dense foods from the nutritional weaklings. The Japanese government, in its nutrition advice, recommends that people consume no fewer than 30 different foods each day! Finally: Mix up your diet from day to day. You'll be assured of getting more of the nutrients you need by eating one mix of nutritionally dense foods today, and a different mix tomorrow.

Eating with Nutrient Density in Mind

Choosing nutrient-dense foods gives you the most nutrition bang for your calorie buck—which is the secret to great health and a healthy body weight. Here are some examples that illustrate the three dimensions of nutrient density.

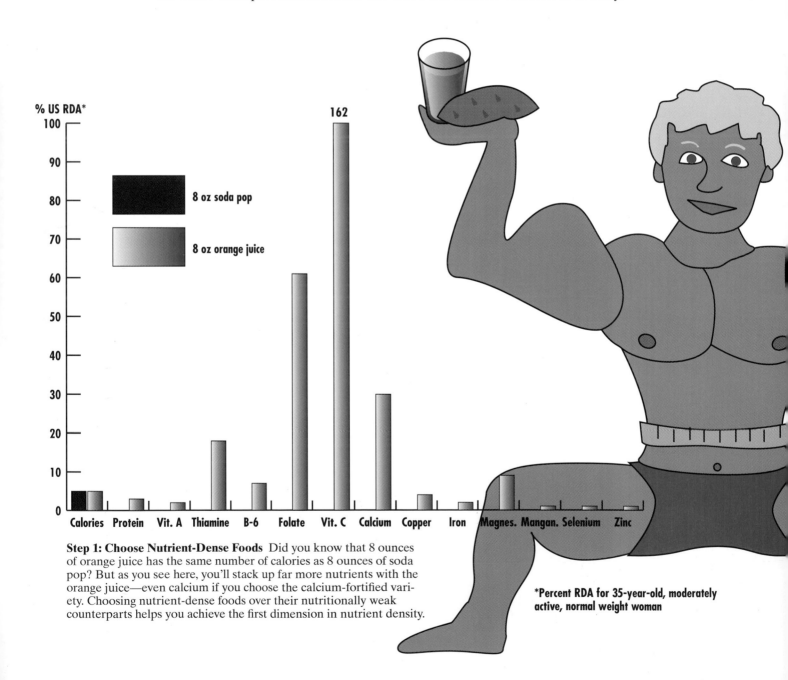

% US RDA*

Legend:
- 8 oz soda pop
- 8 oz orange juice

Vit. C: 162

X-axis labels: Calories, Protein, Vit. A, Thiamine, B-6, Folate, Vit. C, Calcium, Copper, Iron, Magnes., Mangan., Selenium, Zinc

Step 1: Choose Nutrient-Dense Foods Did you know that 8 ounces of orange juice has the same number of calories as 8 ounces of soda pop? But as you see here, you'll stack up far more nutrients with the orange juice—even calcium if you choose the calcium-fortified variety. Choosing nutrient-dense foods over their nutritionally weak counterparts helps you achieve the first dimension in nutrient density.

***Percent RDA for 35-year-old, moderately active, normal weight woman**

Step 2: Don't Dilute Your Nutrients with Empty Calories Grabbing a bag of chocolate candies—or some other high calorie, low nutrient item—dilutes the nutrients you've already eaten. Just one bag of chocolate candies uses up at least 10% of your calorie allotment for the day, without bolstering your nutrient density. Every time you make a food choice, ask yourself if the item you're about to choose is nutrient dense or just empty calories—and forgo the latter.

Step 3: Choose Many Different Nutrient-Dense Foods To achieve this third dimension in nutrient density, don't choose the same nutrient-dense foods—or even the same combination—day after day. Choose lots of different nutritionally dense foods today, and a different mix tomorrow. Here, see how more nutrients pile higher when you achieve this goal. Try to choose at least 10 to 15 different nutrient-dense foods daily to stack up a good complement of most nutrients.

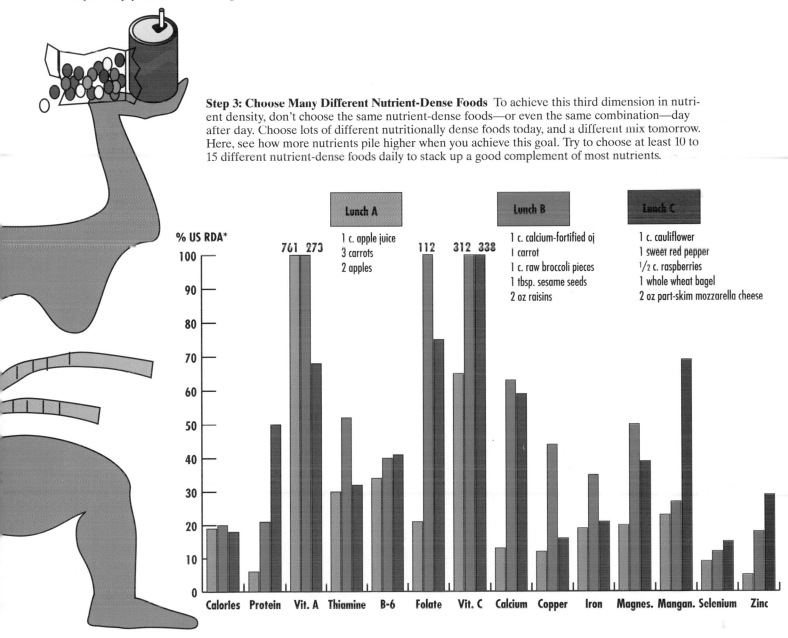

Lunch A
1 c. apple juice
3 carrots
2 apples

Lunch B
1 c. calcium-fortified oj
1 carrot
1 c. raw broccoli pieces
1 tbsp. sesame seeds
2 oz raisins

Lunch C
1 c. cauliflower
1 sweet red pepper
½ c. raspberries
1 whole wheat bagel
2 oz part-skim mozzarella cheese

% US RDA*

761 273   112 312 338

Calories Protein Vit. A Thiamine B-6 Folate Vit. C Calcium Copper Iron Magnes. Mangan. Selenium Zinc

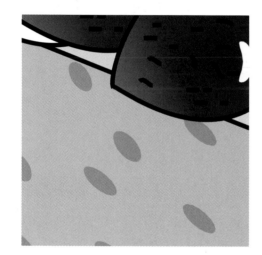

How to Devise a Low-Fat Diet—and Stick to it

ARE YOU ONE of those people who, by the light of day, eats what you think you should eat—a diet devoid of fat? And then, with stomach growling and taste buds hankering for *real* food at night, you dip into—and devour—a pint of death-by-chocolate premium ice cream, a bag of chips and dip, or some other high-fat item?

You're not alone. Tracking—and slashing—fat grams rates right up there with the most popular nutrition crazes of the 1990s. While it's a laudable goal and a sound health maneuver, we've carried it so far that many people are in a yo-yo situation: They go totally fat free all day, or perhaps a few days at a time, and then end up binging on one or a combination of high-fat foods. As a result, many Americans still eat too many calories as fat: On average, Americans eat 34% of calories as fat, when it would be much healthier to limit fat to a maximum of 30% of calories, or less.

In this chapter, you'll learn how to set a healthy fat intake, how to use low-fat products appropriately, and how to devise a low-fat diet that you can follow for the rest of your life. And because so many of us rely on convenience foods, you'll also learn how to use the new food label to track fat grams. Remember the ultimate rule: If you don't like the food you're eating, or if you constantly feel deprived, you won't stick with even the most carefully crafted low-fat diet.

Contrary to what you may have been led to believe, everyone does need fat to live (see Chapter 3). While you only need about 20 grams per day, it's almost impossible to limit yourself to such a paltry amount. Instead, try to limit your fat to a maximum of 30% of your day's calorie allowance. Before you translate that into fat grams, you'll need to know that each gram of fat has 9 calories (fats are the most compact source of calories). Now, here's how to do the math. Multiply your daily calorie allowance by 30%, which gives you the number of calories as fat you should eat in a day. Then divide the number of fat calories by 9 to determine the number of fat grams you should eat in a day.

Here's an example of how to make those calculations, using an average, normal-weight woman aged 30 who should eat about 2,000 calories each day. Multiply 2,000 calories by 30%; this equals 600 calories as fat. Then divide 600 calories by 9; this equals 67 grams of fat.

Realistically, you might want to use a sliding scale of fat intake: Some days trim your fat down to 20% of your daily calorie intake, other days go up to 30%, and still others slide in somewhere in between. Building in this flexibility is not only more realistic, it also has a psychological bonus: If you think you're still within an acceptable range, you're more apt to feel successful at eating healthy amounts of fat. Aiming for the lower intake, on the other hand, may set you up for feeling like a failure on the days you're higher than 20% but actually still within a healthy range.

While many of us have the best intentions of eating only wholesome foods made from scratch, such a commendable goal just isn't realistic in our fast-paced, mobile society. Instead, set another goal to choose *healthier* fast and convenience foods when that's what your schedule demands. One of your most helpful tools is the *new food label*, which you can identify by its heading *Nutrition Facts*. The new food label was mandated by the government in late 1993; all products had to carry it by May 1994. Refer to the diagram on the following pages for help in deciphering the many helpful facts it contains.

There's one point that deserves repeating here: Pay attention to serving size. Labels list fat grams for a *specific* serving size. In some cases, a package that appears to be one serving size to you may actually be labeled as 2 or 3 servings. Eating the whole package, then, means you'd get 2 or 3 times the fat listed for one serving. The bottom line is that serving up the portion indicated on the label (or calculating your fat intake according to what you've actually eaten) is key to tracking fat grams accurately.

In many cases, low- or nonfat products can add new dimensions to your dinner plate: Rather than foregoing sour cream for your baked potato, you can top it with a generous scoop of the nonfat alternative; rather than refuse your craving for tortilla chips, you can grab a handful of the nonfat variety.

But let's face it. Too many times our food choices are driven by two disparate factors: how we want our clothes to fit, and what our taste buds demand. These competing desires set up a vicious cycle: People skimp all day and then turn to fake foods—artificially sweetened, no-fat desserts loaded with the flavors they crave. Because a product like a box of cookies has a no-fat label, some people feel free to eat a whole box. But there are at least two problems with this practice: These products are almost devoid of nutrients, and they still can be surprisingly high in calories. While one nonfat cookie at 60 calories is an acceptable treat, a box of 20 quickly rings up 1,200 extra calories. On top of that, the cycle isn't complete. Still craving fat, many people go on to consume some high-fat item anyway.

Instead of using nonfat desserts to make up for the flavors you haven't gotten be-cause you've skimped all day, use them instead as substitutes for higher fat desserts—after first eating the healthy diet we've described in earlier chapters. Enjoy one or two lowfat cookies or a modest-sized bowl of nonfat frozen yogurt. Think of these items as the icing on the cake—where the cake is actually the healthy food you need to fuel your body for maximum performance.

When using other nonfat products, make sure you like both the taste and texture. Nonfat cheese, for example, just doesn't make the grade for many people. So, rather than settle for it and then later raid the refrigerator for something more satisfying, choose what will satisfy you the first time around. Try the lower-fat versions, or just less of the high-fat version you truly love. In many cases, a progressive switch to the lowest-fat version works best in the long run. If you're currently using whole milk, for exam-ple, switch first to 2%, then to 1%, and finally to ½% or skim milk.

Encouragingly, research has proven that people who trim the fat from their diets in a wise and moderate way end up preferring a lighter style of eating. Lowfat-eating converts find that they feel physically uncomfortable after splurging on a higher-fat meal. This is probably due to two factors: Fat delays the emptying of the stomach, which makes you feel stuffed longer. Also, some researchers believe that people de-velop an aversion to the taste and texture of fatty foods because they learn to associate these characteristics with not feeling well. Finally researchers believe that the longer a person follows a wise low-fat eating plan, the greater is his or her success of sticking to it for life.

One final note: Don't forget what you've learned in earlier chapters. Limit satu-rated fat intake, trying to use poly- and monounsaturated fats for as many as your fat grams as possible (see also Chapter 13).

How to Use the New Food Label to Track Fat Grams

Prepackaged foods come in handy for busy schedules. Learning how to choose them and use them appropriately puts you ahead of the pack in tracking and limiting fat grams. Here's how to use the pertinent points on labels.

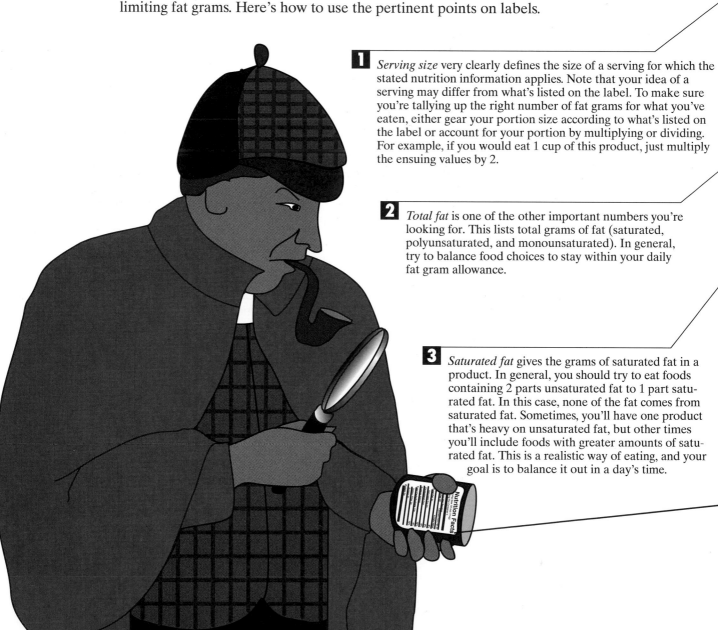

1 *Serving size* very clearly defines the size of a serving for which the stated nutrition information applies. Note that your idea of a serving may differ from what's listed on the label. To make sure you're tallying up the right number of fat grams for what you've eaten, either gear your portion size according to what's listed on the label or account for your portion by multiplying or dividing. For example, if you would eat 1 cup of this product, just multiply the ensuing values by 2.

2 *Total fat* is one of the other important numbers you're looking for. This lists total grams of fat (saturated, polyunsaturated, and monounsaturated). In general, try to balance food choices to stay within your daily fat gram allowance.

3 *Saturated fat* gives the grams of saturated fat in a product. In general, you should try to eat foods containing 2 parts unsaturated fat to 1 part saturated fat. In this case, none of the fat comes from saturated fat. Sometimes, you'll have one product that's heavy on unsaturated fat, but other times you'll include foods with greater amounts of saturated fat. This is a realistic way of eating, and your goal is to balance it out in a day's time.

Nutrition Facts

Serving Size 1/2 cup (114g)

Serving Per Container 4

Amount Per Serving

Calories 90 | Calories from Fat 30

% Daily Value*

Total Fat 3g | **5%**

Saturated Fat 0g | **0%**

Cholesterol 0mg | **0%**

Sodium 300mg | **13%**

Total Carbohydrate 13g | **4%**

Dietary Fiber 3g | **12%**

Sugars 3g

Protein 3g

Vitamin A	80%	•	Vitamin C	60%
Calcium	4%	•	Iron	4%

* Percent Daily Values are based on a 2,000 calorie diet. Your daily values may be higher or lower depending on your calorie needs:

	Calories	2,000	2,500
Total Fat	Less than	65g	80g
Sat Fat	Less than	20g	25g
Cholesterol	Less than	300mg	300mg
Sodium	Less than	2,400mg	2,400mg
Total Carbohydrate		300g	375g
Fiber		25g	30g

Calories per gram:

Fat 9 • Carbohydrate 4 • Protein 4

4 *Calories from fat* is another piece of information that helps you judge a product's nutritional value. If the majority of the calories come from fat, you'll want to include that food cautiously. For example, if you were choosing a frozen dinner for a busy night, select one that has no more than ⅓ of the total calories from fat.

5 *% Daily value* is one of the more confusing pieces of information on the new food label. These values tell you how much of a day's recommended amount for certain nutrients are contained in a serving of that food for someone who needs 2,000 calories per day. Even if you're not aiming for a caloric intake of 2,000 you can use the daily value information to get a general idea of the food's nutritional content.

How to Make Over Meals to Eat Less Fat

The secret in sticking to a lowfat diet is eating food you enjoy. Here Miles performs a make-over on several plates of food, showing you how and where to trim the fat to still leave maximum flavor.

Before

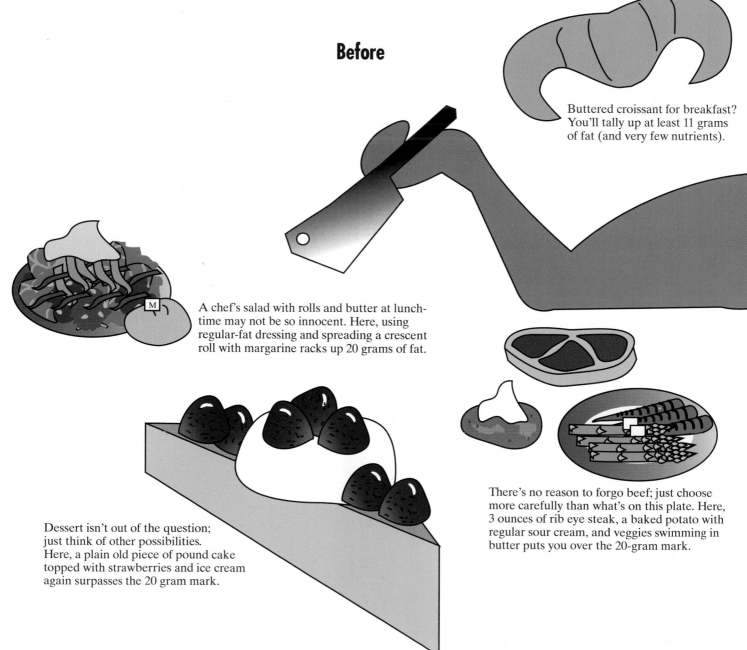

Buttered croissant for breakfast? You'll tally up at least 11 grams of fat (and very few nutrients).

A chef's salad with rolls and butter at lunchtime may not be so innocent. Here, using regular-fat dressing and spreading a crescent roll with margarine racks up 20 grams of fat.

Dessert isn't out of the question; just think of other possibilities. Here, a plain old piece of pound cake topped with strawberries and ice cream again surpasses the 20 gram mark.

There's no reason to forgo beef; just choose more carefully than what's on this plate. Here, 3 ounces of rib eye steak, a baked potato with regular sour cream, and veggies swimming in butter puts you over the 20-gram mark.

After

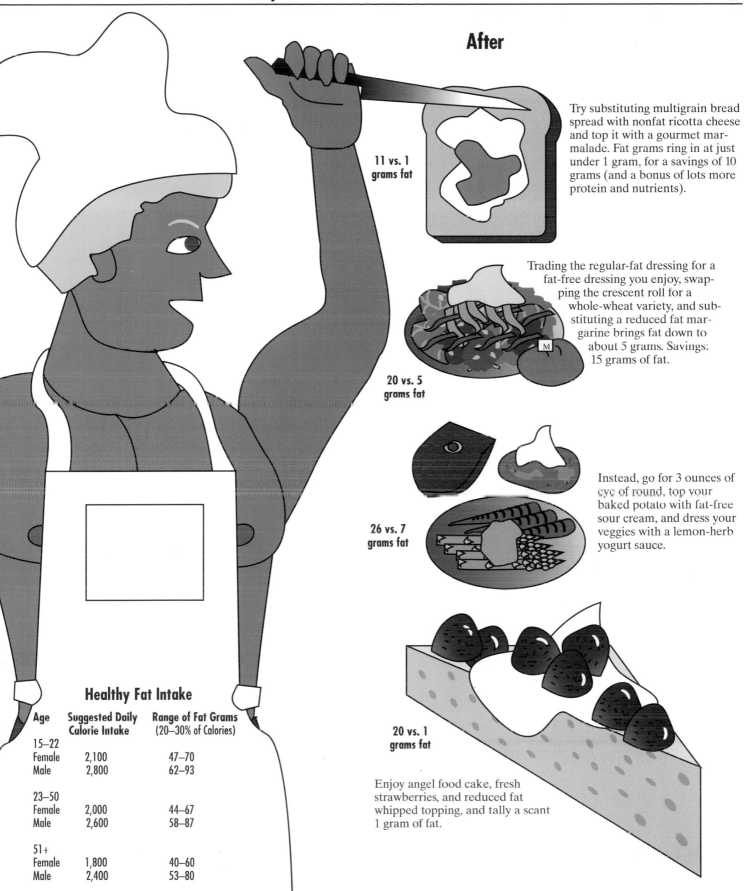

11 vs. 1 grams fat

Try substituting multigrain bread spread with nonfat ricotta cheese and top it with a gourmet marmalade. Fat grams ring in at just under 1 gram, for a savings of 10 grams (and a bonus of lots more protein and nutrients).

Trading the regular-fat dressing for a fat-free dressing you enjoy, swapping the crescent roll for a whole-wheat variety, and substituting a reduced fat margarine brings fat down to about 5 grams. Savings: 15 grams of fat.

20 vs. 5 grams fat

Instead, go for 3 ounces of eye of round, top your baked potato with fat-free sour cream, and dress your veggies with a lemon-herb yogurt sauce.

26 vs. 7 grams fat

20 vs. 1 grams fat

Enjoy angel food cake, fresh strawberries, and reduced fat whipped topping, and tally a scant 1 gram of fat.

Healthy Fat Intake

Age	Suggested Daily Calorie Intake	Range of Fat Grams (20–30% of Calories)
15–22		
Female	2,100	47–70
Male	2,800	62–93
23–50		
Female	2,000	44–67
Male	2,600	58–87
51+		
Female	1,800	40–60
Male	2,400	53–80

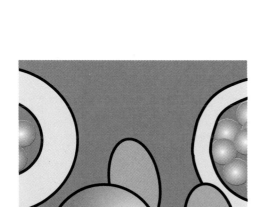

CHAPTER 13

How to Eat to Lower Cholesterol: Fact and Fad

THERE IS A lot of talk these days about cholesterol, heart disease, and diet. Perhaps you find it all a bit confusing—high and low and "good" and "bad" cholesterol, cholesterol in your food and cholesterol in your blood. It's also hard to know what to do about it. Will your heart be healthier if you load up on garlic, olive oil, oat bran, psyllium, walnuts, and red wine? What about vitamin E or a trilogy of B vitamins? In this chapter, we'll help you understand cholesterol once and for all, and we'll focus on how you can eat to lower your cholesterol for the healthiest heart.

While diet is decisively important to your heart's health, no one substance is the magic bullet that will shoot down your risk of heart disease. In fact, even downing a concoction of all of the above "miracle" substances could not erase the effects of one, let alone more than one, poor health habit such as eating too many calories or too much fat, carrying around too much weight, or failing to exercise.

The basic recipe for a heart healthy diet is none other than the basic healthy eating plan you've learned to build in the earlier chapters of this book (especially Chapter 4): lots of complex carbohydrates, a little protein (including red meat!), and a little fat (of the right variety). On the next few pages, we'll look at some of the other substances commonly promoted as heart disease preventives. But first, let's take a closer look at cholesterol and your heart.

Your heart is a strong, muscular pump that beats about 100,000 times each day to send oxygen-rich blood through your arteries to every tissue and cell of the body. Without oxygen, tissues and cells would wither up and die. Just like any other tissue of the body, the heart itself needs plenty of oxygen-rich blood to pump efficiently.

Atherosclerosis, the most common type of heart disease, is characterized by decreased blood flow to the heart. This happens when fatty substances called plaque attach to the inside of arteries, gradually narrowing them. In some cases, plaque buildup becomes so severe that it totally blocks, or *occludes* an artery or arteries. When this happens in the heart's arteries, a heart attack can occur. If vessels supplying blood to the brain are affected, a stroke can occur.

Many factors predict whether or not you'll develop atherosclerosis. In addition to diet, these other factors increase your risk: smoking, high blood pressure, physical inactivity, being overweight, abnormal blood cholesterol levels, and genetics. Fortunately, you can do something about all except the last.

Although the population's blood cholesterol levels have improved since the early 1960s—220 on average then, compared to an average of 205 now—about half of Americans still have elevated cholesterol levels. Lowering cholesterol has indisputable rewards: Lowering a borderline high cholesterol (200–240 milligrams/deciliter, or mg/dl, the unit of measure for reporting blood cholesterol levels) by just 10% (20-24 mg/dl) can slash heart disease risk by 50%. And many people can achieve this sort of drop simply by following a heart-healthy diet. Lowering blood cholesterol readings of above 240 mg/dl yields great benefits, sometimes eliminating the need for costly and often unpleasant cholesterol-lowering drugs.

Blood cholesterol levels are a puzzling matter. Your total cholesterol level is just one piece of the puzzle—and possibly not even the most significant piece. Other numbers, called cholesterol fractions, are more predictive of heart disease risk.

The low-density lipoprotein (LDL)–cholesterol fraction, if too high, increases the risk of plaque depositing in arteries—which is why this fraction is called "bad" cholesterol. The high-density lipoprotein (HDL)–cholesterol fraction is called "good" cholesterol because it tends to protect against plaque depositing in arteries. To minimize heart disease risk, you want your numbers to shape up like this: Total cholesterol should be below 200; LDL-cholesterol should be below 130; and HDL-cholesterol should be above 45. People with a normal total cholesterol level may still be at significant risk of heart disease if their fractions are wrong—if HDL cholesterol is too low or LDL cholesterol is too high. That's why it's important to measure fractions and not just the total number.

Not only are blood cholesterol levels confusing, but cholesterol as a substance is misunderstood. It's little appreciated that the body actually needs cholesterol—it helps form many substances, including skin oils, digestive juices, and vitamin D. In fact, our livers make the overwhelming majority of the body's cholesterol—evidence itself that we need cholesterol to live. It's only when cholesterol levels are too high or in the wrong proportions that we get into trouble.

The picture of your blood fat profile grows yet more confusing when another piece of the puzzle is introduced: triglycerides. Because fat is not soluble in watery blood, it must be transported through the bloodstream packaged in another form, called triglycerides. Unlike cholesterol levels, triglyceride levels are normally higher for several hours after you eat, as fat is digested and moved through the bloodstream as triglycerides to its final destination. That's why your doctor will ask you to not eat for at least 12 hours before checking your triglyceride level. Triglyceride levels that remain high after fasting are not a direct predictor of heart disease risk but may be a clue that a person has an unhealthy diet or has other risk factors for heart disease.

Contrary to popular belief, cholesterol in food is not the most important dietary factor when it comes to raising blood cholesterol levels. In fact, dietary cholesterol is relatively insignificant to your final blood cholesterol reading, as just about 15% of dietary cholesterol is absorbed (the rest simply passes through the intestinal tract unabsorbed). As mentioned above, most of our body's cholesterol is actually made in the liver. Unfortunately, in their battle against blood cholesterol levels, many Americans mistakenly target dietary cholesterol when they should be zeroing in on and reducing intake of another dietary factor: saturated fat.

Saturated fat is indeed the main dietary culprit in raising blood cholesterol levels, both total and LDL. How? In addition to making cholesterol, our liver is responsible for filtering LDL cholesterol from the blood. It does this via thousands of proteins (called LDL receptors) that jut from the surface of each liver cell, snaring LDL particles as they flow by. Saturated fats somehow gum up the works, either by reducing the number of LDL receptors or impairing their efficiency. The result: LDL cholesterol isn't removed, and blood cholesterol levels (both total and the LDL fraction) rise.

On the other hand, unsaturated fats can lower blood cholesterol levels. Monounsaturated fats, such as olive, canola, and peanut oils, selectively lower LDL-cholesterol, while polyunsaturated fats lower both LDL and HDL cholesterol.

But there's another little understood fact about fats and blood cholesterol levels. An overabundance of any type of fat will cause blood cholesterol to rise. That's why you need to think substitution and subtraction when it comes to fats and oils, not addition. In other words, think about reducing all dietary fat and substituting unsaturated for saturated forms.

Incidentally, when you reduce the amount of saturated fat in your diet, you'll also slash cholesterol intake automatically. That's because most foods high in dietary cholesterol are also high in saturated fat (but the reverse is not true).

Overeating, which results in weight gain over time, also raises blood cholesterol levels, especially LDL cholesterol. Exercising, on the other hand, helps raise HDL cholesterol.

Here, along with the facts about them, are some of the substances often thought to prevent heart disease.

Garlic   Affectionately called the "stinking rose," garlic is sold in powder, liquid, and pill forms as a cholesterol-lowering agent; those with stronger stomachs down one or several cloves per day. But can it really lower cholesterol?

The answer is a qualified maybe. While some studies report that the equivalent of one-half to one clove of fresh garlic appears to lower blood cholesterol anywhere from 9% to 20%, the final verdict isn't in. Why? The quality of some of these studies has been deemed questionable. In addition, although garlic is "natural," there isn't sufficient information about garlic's potential to cause problems in large doses—even studies using large doses of garlic involved too few people to detect serious side effects.

The best advice for now? If you like the taste of garlic, use the real thing in your cooking, adding in an extra clove now and then. In fact, if a little more fresh garlic would entice you to eat a vegetable stir-fry, go for it. And until studies prove otherwise, don't throw money into garlic supplements—instead buy those expensive red and yellow bell peppers, stir-frying them with real garlic.

Olive oil   A few years ago when olive oil's ability to lower LDL ("bad") cholesterol hit the news, some restaurants boasted that they were adding olive oil to their dishes. Some people doused food with olive oil, hoping to reap its benefits. But while olive oil and other monounsaturated fats (such as canola oil) do appear to lower LDL cholesterol, there is something fundamentally wrong with the practice of adding olive oil (or any other highly monounsaturated oil) to your diet to decrease your risk of heart disease.

While olive oil is a better fat, it's still a fat. As we said above, monounsaturated fats only work to lower blood cholesterol when *substituted* for saturated fat. And olive oil, like any other fat, still has 120 calories per tablespoon, which quickly breaks anyone's calorie budget and leads to weight gain (which is bad for the heart). So, get out of the "add-in" mode and into the "substitute" mode. Substitute monounsaturated fats like olive oil in all recipes calling for any type of oil or margarine, and cut the total amount whenever possible (learn to stir-fry, for example, with a mixture of olive oil and broth).

Fiber   Two types of fiber, often called *bulk* (see Chapter 15), have received much press for their ability to lower blood cholesterol: psyllium and oat bran. So what's the skinny on their ability to defat the bloodstream?

Psyllium is a high-fiber substance used to make some laxatives. Initial studies suggested that psyllium lowered blood cholesterol, but then experts asked if the effect was simply due to the lowfat diet followed by many psyllium takers. Another round of studies produced good news: Psyllium lowers total blood cholesterol and LDL cholesterol independently of the lowfat diet it may accompany. But to keep a perspective, a lowfat diet still lowers blood cholesterol more than psyllium—about twice as much. The best advice for now: Make a lowfat diet your biggest priority and, if you wish, add 1 to 2 tablespoons of psyllium to your diet daily (this may work especially well for people with high cholesterol levels—it may even delay or eliminate the need for cholesterol-lowering drugs).

Oat bran and other soluble fiber (see Chapter 15 for other good sources of soluble fiber), like psyllium, appear to work independently of a lowfat diet to lower blood cholesterol. Soluble fiber apparently works by "soaking up" cholesterol and removing it from the body. Overall, aim for bulking up your diet with 25–30 grams of fiber each day.

Walnuts (and other nuts)   You may have also read that people who eat more nuts have a lower risk of heart disease. But like olive oil, the nut story is another perfect example of how we should substitute one food for another instead of simply adding in a food like nuts.

Having at least 77% unsaturated fat, nuts are simply a *better* type of fat than other fatty foods (such as cream cheese, butter, and fried snack foods like tortilla chips). The catch: Nuts (like any other fat) are loaded with calories, packing in about 170 calories per ounce (an ounce equals just 2–3 teaspoons). If you eat nuts to lower cholesterol but gain weight because of adding in too many calories, you'll have wiped out any positive effect of the better fat in nuts—you'll actually take a giant step backwards. So, if you like nuts, substitute them for other fats in your diet.

Red wine   Do we have a lesson to learn from the wine-drinking French? Can a glass of burgundy or port now and then actually cleanse the arteries of that gummy, fatty mess called plaque? Indeed, population-based studies have shown repeatedly that people who drink moderate amounts of alcohol have lower rates of heart disease (actually, it doesn't have to be red wine—any alcohol seems to work). The reason: Alcohol seems to raise HDL levels, and preliminary research indicates alcohol helps thin the blood to prevent clot formation. Men experience this benefit with two drinks a day, women with just one (a drink equal 1½ ounces of hard liquor, 12 ounces of beer, or 5 ounces of wine). But go easy: Excessive alcohol consumption is a risk factor for alcoholism, and can also lead to weight gain. If you don't drink now, don't start just to raise your HDLs. A brisk walk can reap the same benefit—and many more.

Vitamin E capsules   Should you take vitamin E to protect against heart disease? As you read in Chapter 7, maybe. The final word isn't in yet; nor do we know if taking large doses of vitamin E over a long period of time can cause ill effects. If you want to take vitamin E, make it a lower priority than eating a lowfat diet, maintaining a trim waistline, and exercising. Also, just to be on the safe side, stick to the lower suggested dose for now, 100 International Units (I.U.).

A trilogy of B vitamins   The role of B-6, folate, and B-12 in preventing heart disease is just emerging, but is quickly gaining momentum. These vitamins apparently work together to keep levels of another substance naturally present in the body, homocysteine, at a healthy low level. This is important, as abnormally high levels of homocysteine apparently contribute to the artery clogging process. But don't head for the vitamin shelf of your drug store or your local health food store. Just be sure to harvest enough of these vitamins by eating your recommended servings of grains, vegetables, and meat.

When it comes to your heart, your first dietary priority is to eat a diet high in complex carbohydrates and low in fat (especially saturated fat). When you do, you'll have a much better chance of achieving the second priority—maintaining a lean body weight, which is key to a healthy heart. Remember, even eating too much complex carbohydrate can lead to heart disease if you eat so much that you gain weight. Garlic, vitamin E, and alcohol may give you an extra edge (when used in moderation) in staving off heart disease—but will contribute nothing if you're eating a high-fat, calorie-overloaded diet.

Understanding Cholesterol Once and For All

No dietary substance is as misunderstood or as maligned as cholesterol. Most people think of it as synonymous with fat, but it's not a dietary fat at all. It's really a waxy lipid. Here we reveal its life-sustaining secrets.

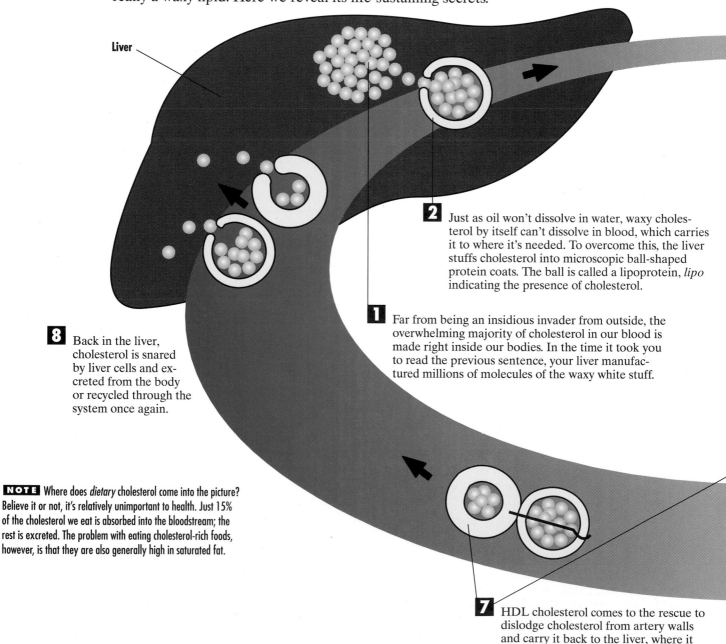

Liver

2 Just as oil won't dissolve in water, waxy cholesterol by itself can't dissolve in blood, which carries it to where it's needed. To overcome this, the liver stuffs cholesterol into microscopic ball-shaped protein coats. The ball is called a lipoprotein, *lipo* indicating the presence of cholesterol.

1 Far from being an insidious invader from outside, the overwhelming majority of cholesterol in our blood is made right inside our bodies. In the time it took you to read the previous sentence, your liver manufactured millions of molecules of the waxy white stuff.

8 Back in the liver, cholesterol is snared by liver cells and excreted from the body or recycled through the system once again.

NOTE Where does *dietary* cholesterol come into the picture? Believe it or not, it's relatively unimportant to health. Just 15% of the cholesterol we eat is absorbed into the bloodstream; the rest is excreted. The problem with eating cholesterol-rich foods, however, is that they are also generally high in saturated fat.

7 HDL cholesterol comes to the rescue to dislodge cholesterol from artery walls and carry it back to the liver, where it can be excreted from the body.

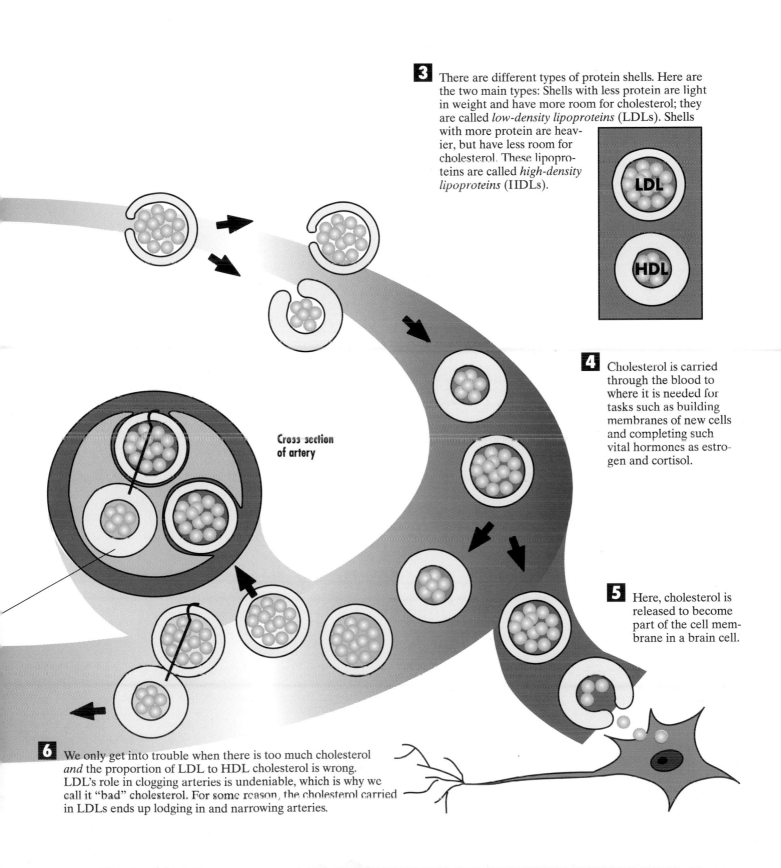

3 There are different types of protein shells. Here are the two main types: Shells with less protein are light in weight and have more room for cholesterol; they are called *low-density lipoproteins* (LDLs). Shells with more protein are heavier, but have less room for cholesterol. These lipoproteins are called *high-density lipoproteins* (IIDLs).

LDL

HDL

4 Cholesterol is carried through the blood to where it is needed for tasks such as building membranes of new cells and completing such vital hormones as estrogen and cortisol.

Cross-section of artery

5 Here, cholesterol is released to become part of the cell membrane in a brain cell.

6 We only get into trouble when there is too much cholesterol *and* the proportion of LDL to HDL cholesterol is wrong. LDL's role in clogging arteries is undeniable, which is why we call it "bad" cholesterol. For some reason, the cholesterol carried in LDLs ends up lodging in and narrowing arteries.

Poly, Mono, and Sat Fats: Not Identical Triplets

Triglycerides, the most common type of fat found in food, can contain any combination of three fatty acids. Dietary fat is named according to the dominant fatty acid. Despite differing by just a couple hydrogen atoms, saturated, monounsaturated, and polyunsaturated fats affect blood cholesterol fractions quite differently. In this picture, each type of dietary fat is placed on its own liver cell, with the bloodstream flowing around all the cells. You can see the effect each type of dietary fat has on blood cholesterol fractions.

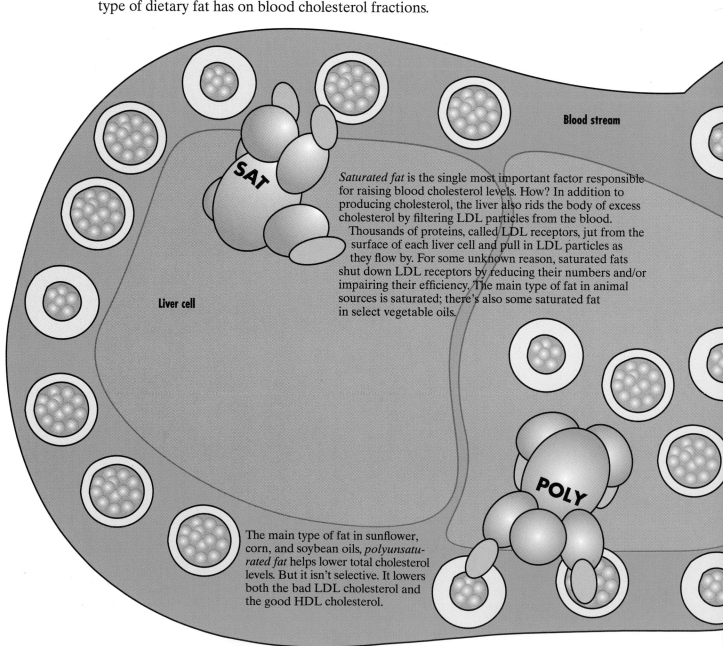

Blood stream

SAT

Liver cell

Saturated fat is the single most important factor responsible for raising blood cholesterol levels. How? In addition to producing cholesterol, the liver also rids the body of excess cholesterol by filtering LDL particles from the blood.

Thousands of proteins, called LDL receptors, jut from the surface of each liver cell and pull in LDL particles as they flow by. For some unknown reason, saturated fats shut down LDL receptors by reducing their numbers and/or impairing their efficiency. The main type of fat in animal sources is saturated; there's also some saturated fat in select vegetable oils.

POLY

The main type of fat in sunflower, corn, and soybean oils, *polyunsaturated fat* helps lower total cholesterol levels. But it isn't selective. It lowers both the bad LDL cholesterol and the good HDL cholesterol.

Two Types of Lipoproteins

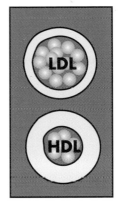

Low-density lipoprotein ("bad" cholesterol)

High-density lipoprotein ("good" cholesterol)

Fish-eating Eskimos taught us another fat lesson: Omega-3 fatty acids, a type of fat found in significant quantities in fish such as salmon and mackerel and in soybean and canola oils, may help fight heart disease. How? By lowering LDL cholesterol and triglyceride levels in the blood. Does that mean fish-oil capsules are a good idea? Probably not, say nutrition experts—stick with the real thing.

MONO

Greeks living on Crete, who consume most of their dietary fat as olive oil, taught us that *monounsaturated fat* (such as that found in olive oil) tends to lower levels of the bad LDL cholesterol, but maintain levels of good HDL cholesterol. Peanut and canola oils also have predominantly monounsaturated fatty acids.

Proportions of Fat in Cooking Oils

Oil	% Sat fat	% Mono fat	% Poly fat
Almond	8	70	18
Avocado	11	71	31.5
Canola	7	58.5	29
Coconut	86.7	6	1.5
Corn	12.5	24	59
Cottonseed	25.7	17.6	52.2
Olive	13.3	73	8.1
Palm	49.2	36.7	9.5
Palm kernel	82	11.7	1.5
Peanut	17	46	31.6
Safflower	8.8	11.7	74
Sesame	13.9	39.7	42
Soybean	14.7	23.5	58
Sunflower	10	19.8	65

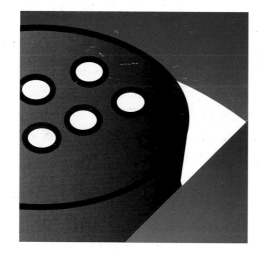

CHAPTER 14

Re-salt Your Diet to Control Blood Pressure

YOU WERE PROBABLY surprised to read the word re-salt in the title of this chapter. No doubt you would have expected *De-salt* Your Diet. But, as you'll see, controlling blood pressure requires more than just cutting out table salt. It also requires adding in the right amounts of other minerals, substances you can think of as health-promoting salts.

Some 50 million Americans, or one of every four adults, have high blood pressure, also called hypertension. It is the single most significant risk factor for stroke and a major contributor to heart disease and kidney failure. Blood pressure is expressed as one number over another. The top number is the *systolic pressure*, or the pressure on arteries as the heart beats, and the bottom number is the *diastolic pressure*, the pressure on arteries between beats of the heart. Someone is said to have hypertension when the blood pressure is at or above 140/90 mm Hg (or millimeters of mercury, the unit for measuring blood pressure).

Eating too much salt is one risk factor for developing hypertension. More precisely, it's the sodium portion of table salt, officially called sodium chloride, that is most responsible for raising blood pressure. There are actually two ways that sodium can raise blood pressure. First, *all* people experience some elevation in blood pressure with too much sodium. In addition, select people are called "salt sensitive." These people are exquisitely sensitive to sodium, and they will experience even greater rises in blood pressure with excessive sodium; they'll also experience more significant drops in blood pressure when dietary sodium is reduced. Some 30–50% of people with hypertension are salt sensitive, as is a smaller percentage of the general population. Because there is no easy way to determine who is salt sensitive, health experts recommend that everyone moderate sodium intake.

True, the body needs sodium to function normally. It helps balance fluids in the body, working in concert with potassium and other minerals. But when we eat too much sodium, the blood draws in extra fluid to try to dilute that sodium, creating a larger volume of fluid inside arteries than the body needs. The result: The extra volume puts more pressure on arteries, which is reflected in a higher blood pressure reading. A high sodium intake can also cause the body to lose calcium in the urine, increasing a person's risk for osteoporosis.

The average sodium intake in this country is several magnitudes higher than what the body needs. We only require about 200 milligrams (mg) of sodium daily, and the average intake is a whopping 4,000 to 6,000 mg. Experts say that limiting sodium to 2,400 mg would help significantly in reducing blood pressure. And lowering systolic blood pressure (the top number) by just 3 mm Hg could decrease the number of deaths due to stroke by 8% and the number of heart disease deaths by 5%.

Limiting sodium, however, is more difficult than just passing up the salt shaker at the table. That's because sodium, in many different forms, is used to process, flavor, and preserve foods. Among these other forms of sodium are sodium caseinate, monosodium glutamate, trisodium phosphate, sodium ascorbate, sodium bicarbonate, and sodium stearoyl lactylate.

Fortunately, the new food labels (which became mandatory in May 1994), make it easier to scout out high sodium foods. The new labels list the actual number of sodium milligrams per serving. In addition, some foods contain a "descriptive" claim on the label. But use foods with these descriptors carefully. Here's why. Some of the descriptive labels give a fairly clear indication of the sodium content of that food, while others are difficult to interpret. Included among those with a clearer definition of the sodium content are the following: *Sodium-free* means less than 5 milligram (mg) per serving of food; *very low sodium* means 35 mg per serving; *low-sodium* means 140 mg or less per serving. Here are a few examples of deceptive sodium descriptors:

Light in sodium or lightly salted. To display this claim, a food must have at least 50% less sodium per serving than the reference food. For example, soy sauce may say "light in sodium" if it has 50% less sodium than the regular product. But such foods could still have a significant amount of sodium. "Light in sodium" soy sauce would still have 384 mg of sodium per tablespoon.

Reduced or less sodium. A food need only have 25% less sodium than the reference food to sport this claim. Using the example of soy sauce, "reduced sodium" soy sauce would still have 576 mg of sodium per tablespoon.

The best advice: Turn immediately to the label's chart to check the exact number of milligrams per serving (however, you're safe with products labeled sodium-free). Also, remember the importance of serving size. Like fat grams, sodium milligrams are listed per serving size as defined by the manufacturer. If you eat more or less than the indicated serving size, calculate up or down.

The good news is that if you're eating the type of diet described in this book—a diet loaded with fruits, vegetables, and whole grains—you'll be limiting dietary sodium automatically. As they come from nature, most foods are naturally low in sodium. Short of tallying sodium intake, here are general guidelines that will help limit sodium intake: Avoid processed and convenience foods when possible, choosing instead foods as they come from nature (fruits, vegetables, and whole grains). When you use convenience and processed foods, check out the label. Try to choose items that have no more than 140–200 milligrams per serving, or if you're choosing a whole convenience meal (such as a frozen dinner), try to stay around 500–1,000 milligrams. Use processed meats, such as luncheon meats, sausages, and bacon, occasionally rather than regularly. Choose fresh or frozen vegetables over canned; if you used canned, buy sodium-free varieties or rinse. Buy plain pastas and add your own spices rather than buying packaged pasta mixes. Use the salt shaker sparingly when cooking food, and try not to use it at the table. If you're tempted by the salt shaker, simply remove it from the table. Replace it with shakers of pepper or an herb combination, or try using a little lemon juice. Replace garlic salt, onion salt, and the like with powders. Leave out some or all of the salt when baking (but this doesn't work in recipes calling for yeast, as salt controls the rate of yeast fermentation and therefore the texture of your finished product).

So far, we've only talked about de-salting your diet. Here's the other part of the equation: re-salting your diet. At least three other minerals are important in controlling blood pressure: potassium, magnesium, and calcium. We know from many research studies that hypertension is much more common in people whose intake of potassium is low. Increasing potassium, according to researchers, can actually lessen the need for hypertension medication (but don't change your medication schedule without consulting your physician). By some estimates, potassium appears to be 2½ times as effective at lowering blood pressure as the same amount of sodium is at raising it. (But that doesn't give you license to hit the salt shaker heavily.) Although there is no recommended dietary allowance for potassium, the National Academy of Sciences suggests 2,000 mg per day for adults. As you'll note on the pages that follow, many of the foods high in potassium are the same foods that are high in vitamins and minerals! Magnesium and calcium are also key in reducing blood pressure, so be sure to get plenty of these nutrients as well.

A bit of other advice to keep blood pressure low: Get plenty of exercise (at least 20 minutes 3 times per week. Maintain a healthy body weight (weight loss has a far greater blood pressure–reducing effect than salt restriction). And if you drink alcohol, do so in moderation.

How Sodium and Other Minerals Affect Blood Pressure

Sodium, one ingredient of table salt, can raise blood pressure when consumed in excessive quantities. Other minerals—potassium, chloride, and magnesium among them—help lower blood pressure. Here's how they work in the body to influence blood pressure.

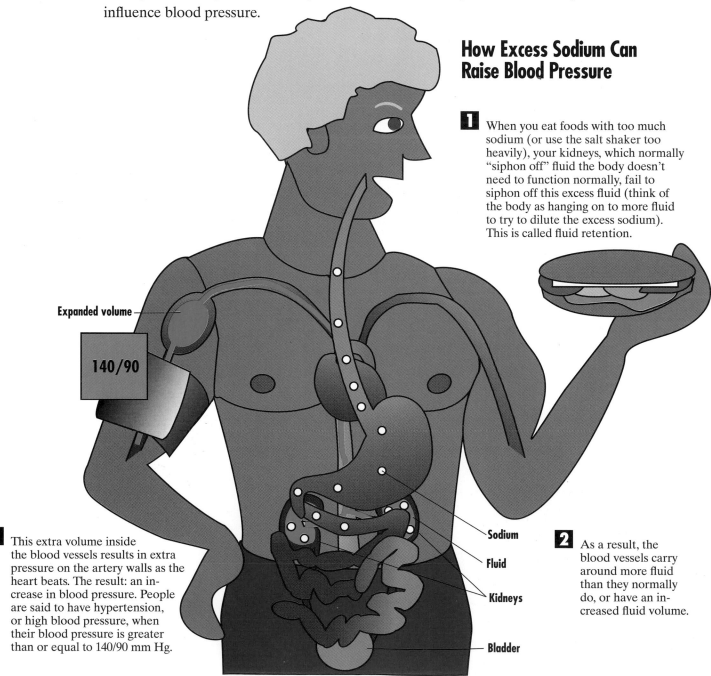

How Excess Sodium Can Raise Blood Pressure

1 When you eat foods with too much sodium (or use the salt shaker too heavily), your kidneys, which normally "siphon off" fluid the body doesn't need to function normally, fail to siphon off this excess fluid (think of the body as hanging on to more fluid to try to dilute the excess sodium). This is called fluid retention.

2 As a result, the blood vessels carry around more fluid than they normally do, or have an increased fluid volume.

3 This extra volume inside the blood vessels results in extra pressure on the artery walls as the heart beats. The result: an increase in blood pressure. People are said to have hypertension, or high blood pressure, when their blood pressure is greater than or equal to 140/90 mm Hg.

Expanded volume

140/90

Sodium

Fluid

Kidneys

Bladder

How Other Minerals Can Lower Blood Pressure

1 Magnesium most likely helps keep blood pressure at a normal low reading by moderating the strength of the contractions on the artery walls.

3 Potassium may exert more than one effect on the body to lower blood pressure.

2 Calcium helps lower blood pressure by much the same mechanism as potassium: It acts like a diuretic and also helps keep artery walls from contracting too strongly.

120/80

4 We know for a fact that potassium acts somewhat like a diuretic, or substance that helps the body flush out extra fluid. When fluid levels are normal or there is no fluid retention, there is a greater chance that blood pressure will be normal.

5 Potassium may also help keep artery walls relaxed. Relaxed arterial walls do not contract as strongly as more "taut" or rigid arterial walls, which means the pressure created with each heart beat is not as great. The result: Blood pressure is lower.

How to Re-Salt Your Diet to Lower Blood Pressure

Without a doubt, a diet high in sodium raises blood pressure. In addition to lowering dietary sodium, you can lower your blood pressure by re-salting your diet with plenty of other minerals. Just as the two minerals sodium and chloride make up ordinary table salt, think of combining these other important blood pressure-lowering minerals as other salts to help you achieve a healthy low blood pressure reading.

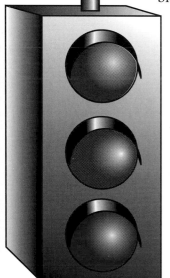

⊖ **Subtract High Sodium Foods**

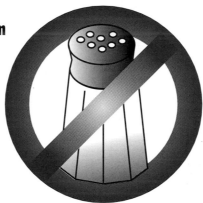

1 Remove the salt shaker from your table, and try to salt food only lightly (or not at all during cooking). Surprisingly, though, salt from the salt shaker is not even the most significant source of sodium for most people. Check out some other surprising sources of sodium.

2 How much salt is in your salt substitute? Are you using products like garlic salt, onion salt, and monosodium glutamate to try to avoid sodium? After seeing how high many are in sodium, try some of the alternatives listed here.

Salt Substitute	Sodium (mg/tsp.)	Alternative	Sodium (mg/tsp.)
Quick chili seasoning	165	Chili powder	0–25
Garlic salt	1,300	Garlic powder	1
Onion salt	1,300	Onion powder	1
Seasoned salt	1,300	Herbs	0
Lite salt	1,100	Herbs or salt sub.	0
Seasoning blends	300–1,400	Herbs or salt sub.	0

3 Are you surprised to find salt hiding here?

Food	Sodium (mg/serving)
Canned soups	800–1,200/1 cup
Healthy Choice or *Special Request* canned soups	400–500/1 cup

Fast Food	Sodium (mg/serving)
Breakfast Sandwich	700–2,000
Sandwich	500–1,400
Fried chicken	300–800/piece

Food	Sodium (mg/serving)
Luncheon meat	300–500/ounce
Lite luncheon meat	200–400/ounce
Snack foods (chips, etc.)	200–600/ounce (not even a handful!)
Lite frozen dinners	300–1,000/meal

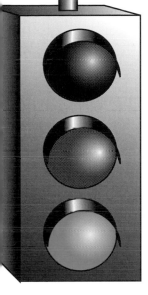

Add Plenty of Other Minerals

4 Add lots of potassium-rich foods. (Always ask your doctor if you can safely pile in lots of potassium-rich foods. Some people, such as those with kidney abnormalities, may tolerate only limited amounts of potassium.) Try for at least 2,000 milligrams of potassium daily. Try these foods containing generous amounts of potassium.

Foods with 300–400 mg Potassium
$\frac{1}{2}$ cup prune juice
$\frac{3}{4}$ cup vegetable juice cocktail (go for the reduced sodium variety)
$\frac{1}{2}$ cup boiled lentils
$\frac{1}{2}$ cup steamed spinach
$3\frac{1}{2}$ ounces baked flounder or sole

Foods with 500–600 mg Potassium
8 ounces low-fat yogurt
10 dates

Foods with 400–500 mg Potassium
1 cup skim milk
1 medium banana
1 cup cantaloupe pieces
$\frac{1}{2}$ cup baked winter squash
$3\frac{1}{2}$ ounces cooked beef tenderloin
3 ounces cooked red snapper

5 Bone up on calcium. Women should aim for no less than 1,500 mg daily, men 800 mg, and youths 1,200 mg. The best sources of calcium are milk and yogurt (300 mg/cup); cheese (100-200 mg/ounce); and calcium-fortified orange juice (200 mg/6 ounces).

Foods with More Than 700 mg Potassium
10 dried apricots
10 dried figs
10 dried prunes
1 medium baked potato with skin

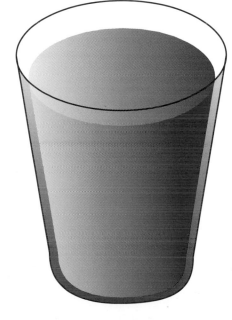

6 Fortify your diet with magnesium. Adults need between 270 and 400 milligrams of magnesium. Good sources of magnesium include many fruits, vegetables, and whole grains. Here are some outstanding examples.

Milk: 30 mg/cup
Oatmeal: 56 mg/cup
Halibut: 90 mg/3 ounces
Whole-wheat bread: 26 mg/slice
Banana: 33 mg/piece
Beets, broccoli, corn: 20 mg/$\frac{1}{2}$ cup
Baked potato with skin: 55 mg/potato

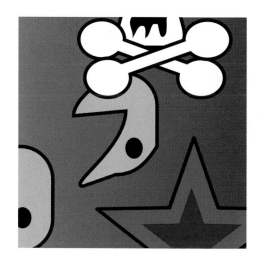

How to Get Enough Fiber to Fight Disease

I F FIBER WERE a true nutrient, it would rate up there with the most underconsumed nutrients in America. Most Americans eat just one-third to one-half the recommended amount of fiber. And the health consequences are both numerous and serious. Indisputable evidence has proven that people who consume enough fiber have lower blood cholesterol levels; lower risk of heart disease, certain cancers, and diseases of the colon; less constipation; and an easier time maintaining a healthy body weight.

As our world has grown more complex, our diets have become more refined: We're eating fewer whole grains, vegetables, and fruits, and replacing such foods with highly refined products. The farther away we get from food as nature made it, the less fiber (and fewer nutrients) we eat. White bread, for example, is a highly stripped-down version of wheat and is consequently very low in fiber (it's also, as we've noted, stripped of many essential vitamins and minerals); white bread generally has 1 gram or less of fiber. A bread made with whole, coarsely ground grains is much higher in fiber (and loaded with essential nutrients!)—whole grain breads have from 2 to 5 grams of fiber per slice. Here's an important connection: High-fiber foods are also high in essential nutrients. You should be noticing as you make your way through this book that a diet that supplies all essential nutrients is also naturally high in fiber, naturally low in fat, and naturally low in salt. That's the beauty of getting all nutrients from real food rather than supplements!

Fiber is found in all varieties of fruits, vegetables, and whole grains. Foods high in fiber are called by another name you already know: unrefined, complex carbohydrates—or, as you read in Chapter 1, foods that haven't been processed to simpler carbohydrates. For example, an apple is a complex carbohydrate, but apple juice is a simple, or *refined* carbohydrate.

Here's another way to think of fiber: The fiber in plants is somewhat akin to the fibers or threads that form your clothing. Just as threads give cloth structure, fiber also lends structure and strength to plants. Partly owing to this strength, fibers in fruits and vegetables are indigestible, which means our bodies cannot break them down.

Just as there is more than one type of thread to make cloth, there are many types of fibers found in plants, and they're divided into two main types: soluble and insoluble. *Soluble* fiber dissolves in the watery contents of the gastrointestinal tract to form a gel. Good sources of soluble fiber include oatmeal (precisely, the bran fraction of oats), barley, kidney beans, some fruits, and some vegetables. *Insoluble* fiber, on the other hand, does not dissolve in the intestine's watery milieu, but instead soaks up water (much like a sponge would) to make stools softer and easier to eliminate. Wheat bran, many vegetables, and other whole grains are good sources of insoluble fiber.

There are several ways fiber works to prevent disease and promote good health. The gel formed by soluble fiber traps substances that may cause cancer, as well as by-products in the large intestine that the body could eventually turn into fat and choles-terol. Insoluble fiber, by increasing the weight of the stool, also washes away disease-causing substances in the intestinal tract—not only more of them, but at a much faster rate. Because stools move through the intestinal tract much faster, there is less time for whatever disease-causing substances are left to come into contact with the tissues of the intestinal tract (that's one of the reasons a high-fiber diet is thought to decrease colon cancer risk). Refer to the illustrations on the following pages for more detailed information on how fiber works to fight disease.

Does getting fiber from a supplement—pills, powders, or wafers—offer the same benefits as getting fiber from food? Definitely not! Fiber supplements contain just one type of fiber, when really you're looking for a mix of lots of different types of fiber. In addition, increasing your fiber with supplements places you at risk of mineral defi-ciency. While any type of fiber reduces the absorption of calcium, zinc, iron, and mag-nesium, you generally don't have to worry about becoming deficient when you get your fiber from food. That's because high-fiber foods are also rich in minerals—containing enough to compensate for reduced absorption.

Yet another reason to get fiber from food instead of pills: Not only will you bulk up your diet, but you'll also be getting plenty of other vitamins and minerals you need. Finally, if you're taking a pill or mixing a powder into a liquid, you're not satisfying your desire to chew. That means that you're still looking for something to *chew on*. On the other hand, when you eat high-fiber foods, you're also satisfying that very impor-tant need to chew. And that means you're less likely to eat low-fiber items, many of which are high in fat and calories.

Just as you shouldn't rely on a supplement containing one type of fiber, you shouldn't rely on just one food for your fiber, such as a bran muffin. Instead, choose from a wide variety of fruits, vegetables, and whole grains. You can start getting enough fiber by choosing a breakfast grain or cereal that's high in fiber, settling for one with no less than 3 grams of fiber per serving. Some high-fiber cereals have as much as 15 grams per serving, varieties to rely on if you have a tough time eating enough fruits, vegetables, and whole-grain products. (Be cautious, however, as many high-fiber cereals can also be high in sugar.) Starting your day with a high-fiber cereal has an added benefit: It will suppress your appetite for hours. Studies show that people who eat a high-fiber cereal for breakfast are less hungry during the day and so eat fewer total calories, fat, and sodium.

By the way, step carefully around bran muffins—they're frequently one of those fat land mines we talked about in Chapter 3 (some commercially prepared bran muffins have an astronomical 30 grams of fat and 500–600 calories); the same is true of granola. And don't rely on a food's crunchiness to signal a high fiber content; crunchy foods aren't always high in fiber. Celery and lettuce, two great crunchers, are actually quite low in fiber. Choose grain products carefully: Make sure they're actually made with the whole grain. Bread labeled "wheat bread," for example, probably has no more fiber than bread labeled "white bread." Whole wheat bread, on the other hand, is most likely much higher in fiber (and other nutrients, too!). Also note that cooking doesn't change a food's fiber content.

How much fiber should you get? Aim for a minimum of 20 grams of fiber (from a variety of sources) and a maximum of 35 (some people tolerate much more, say 45–50 grams daily, but many do not). If you've been eating little fiber, bulk up slowly, adding a few more grams every few days. Raising your fiber level quickly can produce uncomfortable symptoms: bloating, gas, and diarrhea. As you increase fiber intake, cut back to a lower intake if you experience these uncomfortable symptoms, and then increase again slowly after the symptoms have subsided. Also drink plenty of fluids, remembering that soaking up fluid is one of the ways fiber works. Not getting enough fluid with your fiber can actually cause problems: The fiber can become hardened in your intestinal tract, causing constipation.

One final thought about fiber: Many people have taken to "juicing," or pulverizing exotic combinations of fruits and vegetables in special little machines. But if you juice up fruits and vegetables, you often throw away the pulp (and vitamins and minerals) that's left, which means you're throwing out the fiber. That's to say nothing of the concentrated source of calories you drink in juiced concoctions. So rather than juicing, go for the whole fruit and the whole vegetable. You'll eat fewer calories and lots more vitamins and minerals, and you'll bulk up on the fiber that helps fight disease.

How Fiber Helps Control Weight

The health benefits of eating enough fiber are many! Here's how fiber helps control weight.

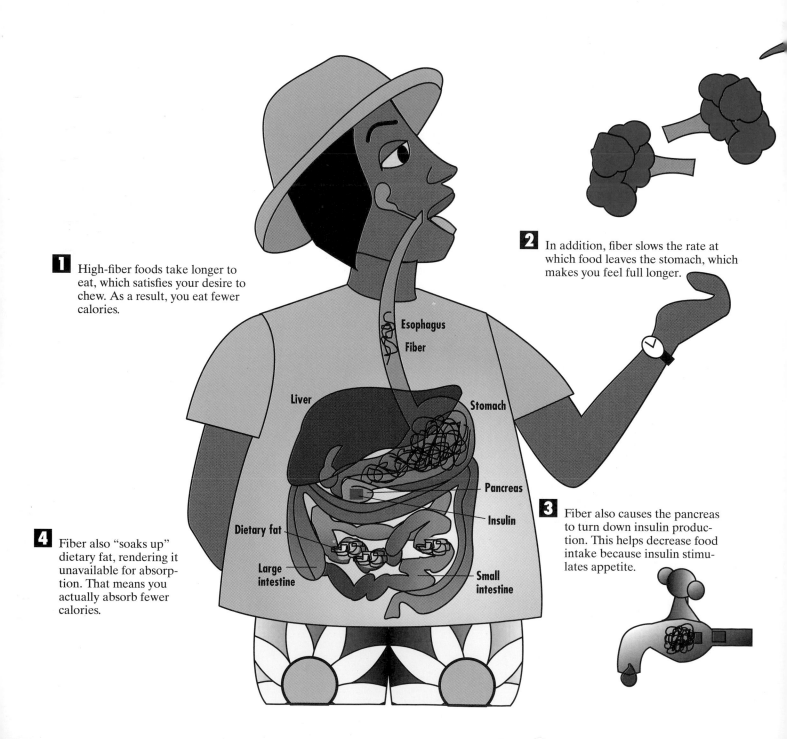

1 High-fiber foods take longer to eat, which satisfies your desire to chew. As a result, you eat fewer calories.

2 In addition, fiber slows the rate at which food leaves the stomach, which makes you feel full longer.

3 Fiber also causes the pancreas to turn down insulin production. This helps decrease food intake because insulin stimulates appetite.

4 Fiber also "soaks up" dietary fat, rendering it unavailable for absorption. That means you actually absorb fewer calories.

Esophagus

Fiber

Liver

Stomach

Pancreas

Insulin

Dietary fat

Large intestine

Small intestine

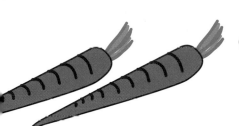
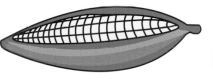
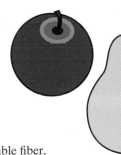

Where the fiber is Some foods are high in soluble fiber, some in insoluble fiber, and some are mixtures. In general, whole grains are highest in insoluble fibers; fruits and vegetables also have some. On the other hand, oats, barley, fruits, vegetables, and legumes are great sources of soluble fiber. The following chart shows how the grams add up.

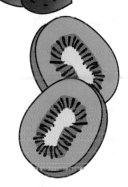

Food (Amount)	Grams Fiber
Broccoli (½ cup)	2.5
Carrots (½ cup)	2.5
Corn (½ cup)	3
Apple (1 medium)	3
Pear (1 medium)	4.5
Strawberries (1 cup)	4
Kiwi (1)	5
Kidney beans (1 cup)	10
Lentils (1 cup)	8
Winter squash (1 cup)	6
Popcorn (3½ cups)	4.5
Figs (2)	4
Orange (1)	4
Spinach (1 cup)	4

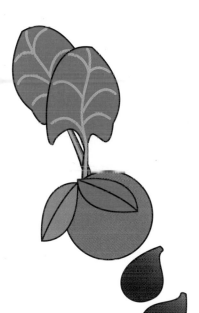
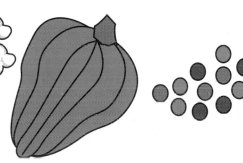
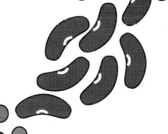

How Fiber Helps Prevent Cancer

People who eat high-fiber diets have a greatly reduced cancer risk. Not only is the risk of colon cancer lower, but so is the risk of breast, prostate, and other cancers throughout the body. Here's how fiber works to prevent cancer.

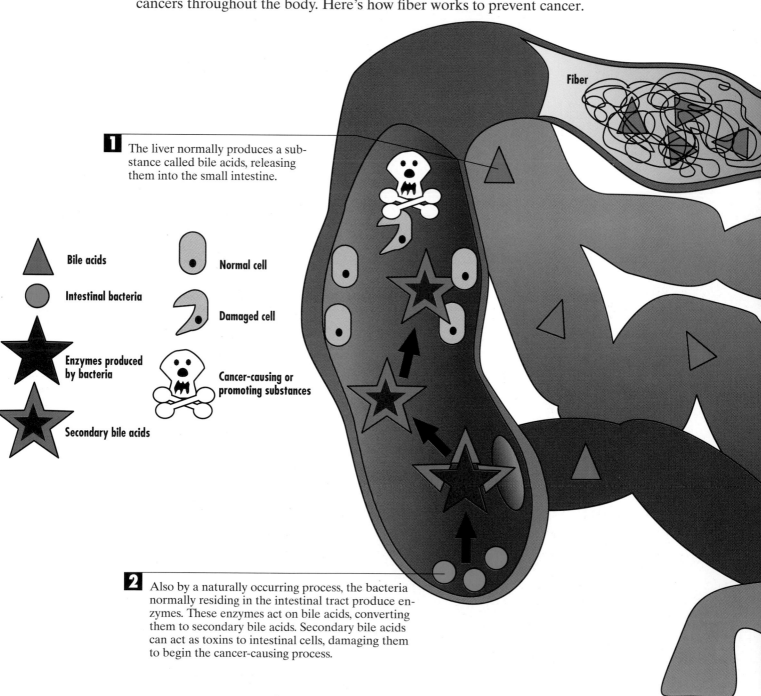

1 The liver normally produces a substance called bile acids, releasing them into the small intestine.

▲ **Bile acids**

● **Intestinal bacteria**

★ **Enzymes produced by bacteria**

★ **Secondary bile acids**

▯ **Normal cell**

◗ **Damaged cell**

☠ **Cancer-causing or promoting substances**

2 Also by a naturally occurring process, the bacteria normally residing in the intestinal tract produce enzymes. These enzymes act on bile acids, converting them to secondary bile acids. Secondary bile acids can act as toxins to intestinal cells, damaging them to begin the cancer-causing process.

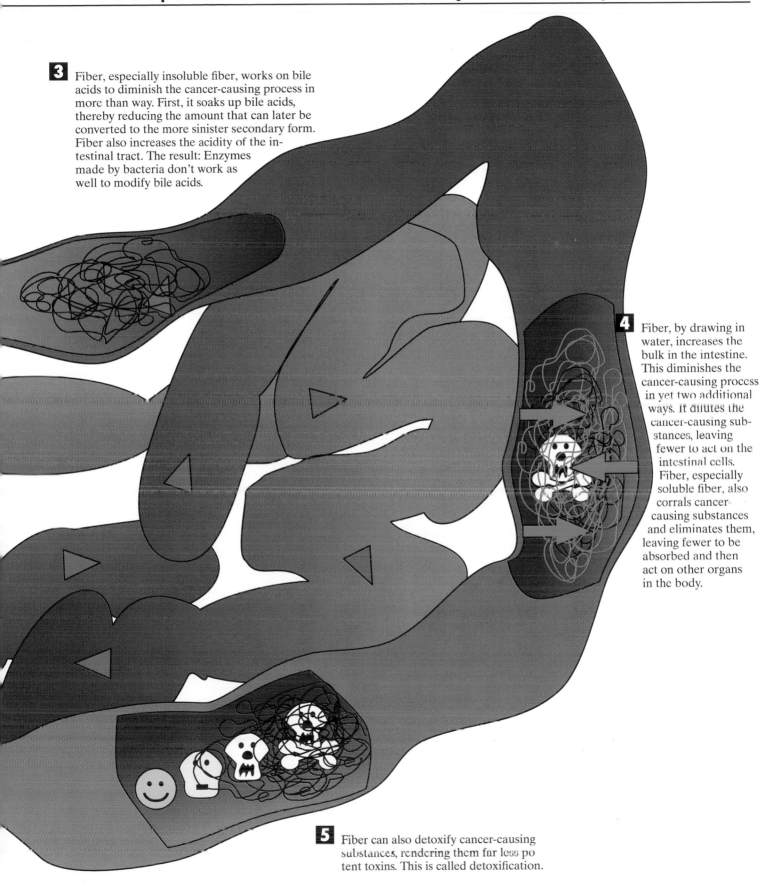

3 Fiber, especially insoluble fiber, works on bile acids to diminish the cancer-causing process in more than way. First, it soaks up bile acids, thereby reducing the amount that can later be converted to the more sinister secondary form. Fiber also increases the acidity of the intestinal tract. The result: Enzymes made by bacteria don't work as well to modify bile acids.

4 Fiber, by drawing in water, increases the bulk in the intestine. This diminishes the cancer-causing process in yet two additional ways. It dilutes the cancer-causing substances, leaving fewer to act on the intestinal cells. Fiber, especially soluble fiber, also corrals cancer-causing substances and eliminates them, leaving fewer to be absorbed and then act on other organs in the body.

5 Fiber can also detoxify cancer-causing substances, rendering them far less potent toxins. This is called detoxification.

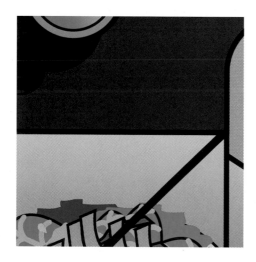

How to Stop Dieting and Be Trim

WHEN IT COMES to weight and food, it's almost as if there is a lapse in reality. Although some two-thirds of American women (as well as an unknown percentage of men) are currently "dieting" or have just finished dieting, the latest health surveys don't reflect these efforts. At least one-third of adults over age 20 are overweight—a weighty 58 million. And they're not just staying heavy—overweight people are growing yet heavier. According to that latest survey, adults weigh, on average, 8 pounds more than they did a decade ago.

Why doesn't this $2-billion-plus effort pay off? Why, even though losing weight is the biggest change most women say they want to make in their lives, aren't they (or men) losing weight? Why are they actually *gaining* weight?

Marie's story tells it all: Battling the 30 pounds she had gradually gained over the course of having three children, Marie went from one weight-loss plan to another. After two weeks on the "jump start" plan offered by a reputable weight-loss program, Marie had lost 8 pounds. But she had also become hungry. The 800-calorie plan had left her ravenous, with a gnawing hunger she gave in to one night when she was tired and frustrated. Feeling guilty about "going off" her "diet," Marie felt defeated and threw in the towel. Over the next few days, she comforted herself with her favorite treats, gaining back the 8 pounds, plus 2 more. Several months later, thinking about her 10-year class reunion, Marie decided to go for the liquid diet routine she had seen on television—two great-tasting shakes early in the day and a regular dinner. That worked for three weeks, but once again, Marie craved real food. In just five days, Marie regained the 9 pounds she had lost, plus 1 more. Soon Marie was 40 pounds, then 50 pounds heavier than she wanted to be. Marie became another dieting casualty.

Marie's is the story of many American dieters—a story of yo-yo dieting. You may have also heard it called skimping and binging (as we said in Chapter 8). People starve themselves for a day or even several days running, successfully dropping a few pounds. But then, starving, they binge and gain those few pounds back. But it's even worse than that: The body has an amazing ability to adjust to these calorie-level yo-yos. Always tuned in to conserving energy, the body slows its metabolic rate when you severely restrict calories, which means that your body doesn't need as many calories, and therefore you don't lose as much as you thought you would. The whole situation is worsened by the *way* you gain back weight. For the most part, you gain back more fat than muscle tissue—which also slows your metabolic rate. That's because fat tissue requires far fewer calories to function than does working muscle tissue.

So what's the way out of this vicious cycle?

Stop dieting and start eating and exercising. Believe it or not, you can reach a healthy body weight without dieting. Remember five six concepts: hunger, appetite, satiety, good health, real food, and exercise.

Many of us confuse hunger and appetite. *Hunger* is that empty-stomach feeling—that growling, gnawing signal your stomach sends to let you know your body truly needs food. *Appetite,* however, is a psychological desire for food. Think of it this way: People who are very ill may go for a day or even days without eating. Although their body needs food, they don't eat because they simply don't have an appetite. On the other hand, how many times have you felt stuffed after a meal but then managed to eat a scrumptious dessert—simply because seeing it whetted your appetite?

And then there's *satiety*, or a feeling of having eaten enough food to satisfy your body's needs. Again, think of stuffing in a dessert on top of an already full stomach—were you miserably uncomfortable for an hour or two after overeating? Recognizing when you're satiated, or physically satisfied, is key to not overeating.

Here's the catch to eating when you're hungry, satisfying your appetite, and not eating anything more when you are satiated: Eat the real food that you enjoy and that satisfies your body's needs for good health. To illustrate, consider what many chronic dieters do: They eat what they consider to be "diet food" all day, but nothing they truly enjoy, nothing that satisfies their appetite. By the light of the moon, however, they eat what they really wanted to have—the food that satisfies their appetite. And because they're physically hungry—if not starving—by the time they finally eat what their appetite demands, they eat beyond the point of satiety and they stuff themselves. Not only do they end up overeating, but they most likely haven't eaten the foods to satisfy their body's needs for good health.

Here's the amazing thing: When you eat real food all day, food that chronic dieters often think of as fattening, you'll no doubt eat fewer calories over the long haul and you'll finally lose weight. By eating a good variety of real food, you'll be satisfying your appetite *and* your hunger *and* your body's needs for good nutrition.

What's more, because you aren't putting your body into a semistarvation state, your metabolism will actually stay higher, which means it will actually be easier to lose weight while eating more food.

Recognize, however, that you're not going to drop 11 pounds the first week, as many programs and fads promise. You may lose 2–3 pounds the first week and then maybe a half to a whole pound each subsequent week; some weeks you may not lose at all. But think about this over the long haul. How many diets have you been on, only to find yourself heavier today than when you started years ago? Wouldn't you rather eat healthy food that you enjoy, avoid that denial-binge cycle, feel strong and energetic, *and* lose weight to boot?

Eating healthy food that satisfies your appetite and your hunger is essential, but there's one piece of the puzzle missing—a very critical piece. *Exercise.* Getting enough exercise is critical for a multitude of reasons. First, you'll burn even more calories than you think. Metabolic rate stays higher for up to 12 hours after exercise, which means you continue to burn more calories in that 12-hour period following exercise than in any other 12-hour period. And if you exercise regularly, your metabolic rate will stay higher for another reason: People who exercise have more muscle tissue than people who don't exercise. As we said above, muscle tissue has a higher calorie requirement than does fat tissue.

In addition, you may actually want to eat less after exercising. Research has proven beyond a shadow of a doubt that exercising squelches your appetite.

The other health benefits of exercising are enormous: Exercise helps raise HDL ("good") cholesterol, helps lower blood pressure, helps diabetics control blood sugar, and helps moderate the stress in your life (which can also help you eat less if you're one of those stress eaters).

Refer to the following pages for more tips on reaching your healthiest weight without dieting.

How to Stop Dieting and Be Trim for Life

It's time to jump out of the dieting cycle that's trapped you for years. Try these suggestions to achieve and maintain a healthy weight.

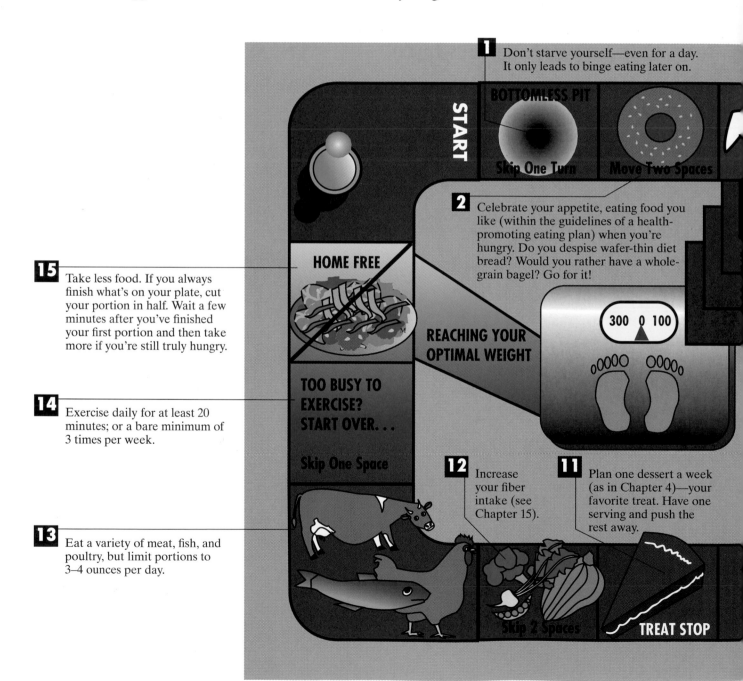

1 Don't starve yourself—even for a day. It only leads to binge eating later on.

BOTTOMLESS PIT
Skip One Turn

Move Two Spaces

START

2 Celebrate your appetite, eating food you like (within the guidelines of a health-promoting eating plan) when you're hungry. Do you despise wafer-thin diet bread? Would you rather have a whole-grain bagel? Go for it!

15 Take less food. If you always finish what's on your plate, cut your portion in half. Wait a few minutes after you've finished your first portion and then take more if you're still truly hungry.

HOME FREE

REACHING YOUR OPTIMAL WEIGHT

300 0 100

14 Exercise daily for at least 20 minutes; or a bare minimum of 3 times per week.

TOO BUSY TO EXERCISE? START OVER. . .

Skip One Space

12 Increase your fiber intake (see Chapter 15).

11 Plan one dessert a week (as in Chapter 4)—your favorite treat. Have one serving and push the rest away.

13 Eat a variety of meat, fish, and poultry, but limit portions to 3–4 ounces per day.

Skip 2 Spaces

TREAT STOP

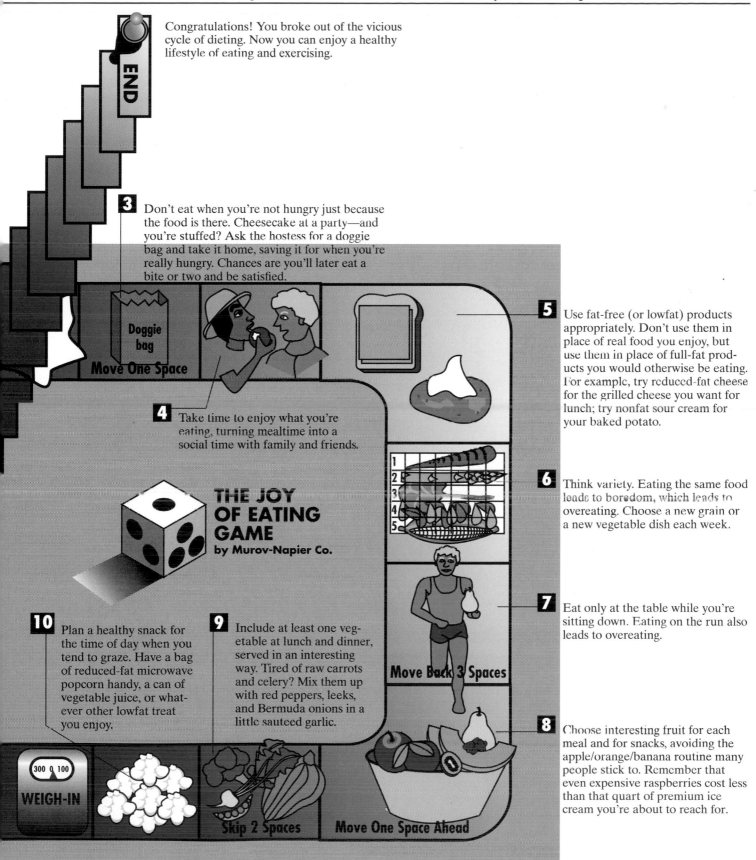

END

Congratulations! You broke out of the vicious cycle of dieting. Now you can enjoy a healthy lifestyle of eating and exercising.

3 Don't eat when you're not hungry just because the food is there. Cheesecake at a party—and you're stuffed? Ask the hostess for a doggie bag and take it home, saving it for when you're really hungry. Chances are you'll later eat a bite or two and be satisfied.

Doggie bag
Move One Space

4 Take time to enjoy what you're eating, turning mealtime into a social time with family and friends.

THE JOY OF EATING GAME
by Murov-Napier Co.

10 Plan a healthy snack for the time of day when you tend to graze. Have a bag of reduced-fat microwave popcorn handy, a can of vegetable juice, or whatever other lowfat treat you enjoy.

9 Include at least one vegetable at lunch and dinner, served in an interesting way. Tired of raw carrots and celery? Mix them up with red peppers, leeks, and Bermuda onions in a little sautéed garlic.

WEIGH-IN   300 0 100

Skip 2 Spaces

Move One Space Ahead

Move Back 3 Spaces

5 Use fat-free (or lowfat) products appropriately. Don't use them in place of real food you enjoy, but use them in place of full-fat products you would otherwise be eating. For example, try reduced-fat cheese for the grilled cheese you want for lunch; try nonfat sour cream for your baked potato.

6 Think variety. Eating the same food leads to boredom, which leads to overeating. Choose a new grain or a new vegetable dish each week.

7 Eat only at the table while you're sitting down. Eating on the run also leads to overeating.

8 Choose interesting fruit for each meal and for snacks, avoiding the apple/orange/banana routine many people stick to. Remember that even expensive raspberries cost less than that quart of premium ice cream you're about to reach for.

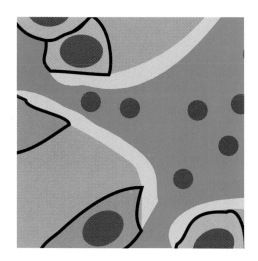

How to Fight Cancer with a Healthy Diet

WOULDN'T IT BE great if you could take a pill to reduce your cancer risk? Many people, in fact, think they can—faithfully washing down their antioxidant tablet with coffee or soda pop. But this is far short of what *really* can be done to mount the best cancer protection defense.

Antioxidants are just part of the cancer protection picture—and there's evidence that antioxidants in food function more effectively than antioxidants in pills (see Chapter 7). It might be the way nature combines antioxidants in food. Or perhaps it's the presence of other naturally occurring substances in food that work in concert with antioxidants to fight off the changes in cells and tissues that lead to cancer. Or maybe it's the fiber in food that helps "soak up" potentially cancer-causing substances. Most likely, though, it's a combination of all these factors—and other factors scientists haven't yet identified.

Cancer strikes about 1.2 million people each year and claims the lives of nearly 540,000. But what is cancer?

Cancer isn't just one disease; it's really a constellation of many similar diseases that are characterized by the uncontrolled growth of abnormal cells. Some substances act on cells to cause changes that lead to this uncontrolled growth, and these substances are called carcinogens. While some carcinogens are identified—tobacco smoke, large doses of radiation, excess sunlight, excess alcohol consumption—many are not. Some substances may become carcinogenic only under certain conditions. It's known, for example, that people who are 40% or more overweight increase their risk of many cancers, including those of the colon, breast, prostate, gallbladder, ovary, and uterus. Also, some substances become more powerful carcinogens in the presences of other substances. Alcohol and tobacco, for instance, cause more cancer in the presence of each other than each does independently. And some people have a greater genetic tendency to develop cancer.

All during our lives, cells throughout our bodies undergo changes—think of them as bumps, bruises, and nicks—that could someday lead to cancer. The more insults cells endure, the greater chance a person has of developing cancer. The goal is to minimize these changes through a healthy lifestyle: avoiding tobacco and excessive sun exposure, limiting alcohol intake, protecting yourself from occupational substances (such as vinyl chloride and asbestos) known to cause cancer, and following a healthy diet. Not only should you start *today* on the path to this healthier lifestyle, but you should also point your children and grandchildren in the right direction. Chances are, the sooner you act to minimize cancer-causing changes, the better your chances are of not getting cancer.

Here's what you need to know about diet to fight off cancer. Various nutrients have been highlighted for their cancer-protection abilities; some are described below. But as you read about them, remember that an increasing body of research points to a diet plentiful in fruits and vegetables in general as being most protective against cancer, as opposed to a diet high in one or another specific nutrient.

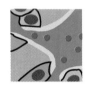

The *antioxidant nutrients* you learned about in Chapter 7 are key to fighting cancer. Vitamins E and C and the carotenes (not only beta-carotene but also alpha-carotene and even other varieties) help stop or reduce the damage to cells caused by free radicals; emerging evidence suggests antioxidants may fight cancer by additional mechanisms. But get them through food, not through pills. You'll find a listing of high-antioxidant foods in Chapter 7.

Selenium is a mineral the body needs to prevent oxidation, the same process that makes butter rancid and metal rust. There is increasing evidence that selenium also helps prevent cancer, but not as an antioxidant. Scientists hot on the trail of selenium's cancer-prevention capabilities think there are at least two ways selenium may fight cancer. First, it may help detoxify, or disarm, carcinogens. It may also induce the death of precancerous cells. Major studies are now underway to help identify how selenium fights cancer as well as how much selenium is necessary. In addition, researchers are trying to determine the best way to administer selenium. While some forms of selenium may quickly become toxic, others do not.

Folic acid, in addition to its roles in keeping red blood cells healthy, making new cells and tissues, and preventing heart disease, plays a role in preventing cancer, especially colon cancer. Scientists think that folic acid somehow ensures that DNA, the recipe by which new cells are made, stays intact to produce an exact, healthy replica. Cells with damaged DNA are far more likely to become cancerous. As with selenium, folic acid experts don't yet know the dose necessary to prevent cancer—but getting at least the RDA is definitely good advice!

Calcium, that great bone builder, may help ward off colon cancer; the same is true for *vitamin D*.

Vitamin A, independently of its precursor carotenes, seems to offer some protection against lung cancer. But remember that it's fat soluble, so consuming too much can be dangerous.

Fiber (also called *dietary bulk)* as you read in Chapter 15, is a very important cancer fighter.

Phytochemicals are the latest food substances identified as cancer warriors (and they may possibly fight off other diseases as well). Scientists speculate that there are thousands of these nonnutrient, naturally occurring substances in plant foods, especially fruits, vegetables, legumes, and some grains. Tomatoes, for example, may have some 10,000 phytochemicals. Current research is now focusing on the mechanisms by which these substances might work against disease. You may be seeing the following phytochemicals in the news: flavonoids (found in citrus fruits, tomatoes, berries, peppers, and carrots), genistein (found in beans, peas, and lentils), indoles (found in broccoli and the cabbage family), isothiocyanates (found in broccoli, cabbage, mustard, and horseradish), lignans (found in flaxseed, barley, and wheat), lycopenes (found in tomatoes and red grapefruit), and triterpenoids (found in citrus fruits).

While the substances you've read about so far help *fight* cancer, another dietary substance actually contributes to *causing* cancer. Excess *dietary fat* seems to be one culprit, especially in causing colorectal cancer (research on fat and breast cancer has failed to find an association). Dietary fat may contribute to the cancer-causing process by increasing the amount of bile acids in the colon. Some researchers think that bile acids are converted to a more sinister form, secondary bile acids, they act as toxins on certain cells, especially cells lining the colon. Although research is inconsistent, it suggests that excess dietary fat may boost breast cancer risk by somehow affecting the level of estrogen in the body, which may promote cancer growth in some women. But these two theories don't totally explain why dietary fat is associated with a higher incidence of cancer. We also know, for instance, that people who consume high-fat diets generally don't eat enough fiber, fruits, or vegetables, and this in itself places people at higher risk of cancer. And we also know that eating too much fat generally translates into eating too many calories. There is increasing evidence that excess calories—of any type—also increase a person's risk for cancer. According to a leading nutrition-cancer researcher, when a person eats too many calories, cancerous cells get the fuel they need to grow. Indeed, animals fed diets designed to keep them lean develop far less cancer than do animals fed diets with a higher calorie content—even when they are exposed to chemicals known to cause cancer.

But let's forget these individual nutrients and food substances and the role they play they in fighting or causing cancer. What does it mean in real food? What exactly should you eat (and not eat) to prevent cancer? You may be surprised to learn that the most powerful cancer-fighting diet is the same diet you've already learned to craft earlier in this book: a diet bursting with fruits, vegetables, and complex carbohydrates, while also being slim on fat, fatty foods, and highly refined items. When you do this, you'll harvest all the nutrients we've talked about that fight cancer, and you'll avoid that slippery substance, fat, which places you at higher risk of cancer and so many other health problems.

This problem deserves repeating: The most convincing evidence about food's ability to fight cancer, in fact, doesn't come from studies of single nutrients or substances. In fact, single-nutrient studies have produced disappointing results when it comes to preventing cancer. Consistently, studies from research centers around the world find that the best cancer protection comes from a diet high in different types of fruits and vegetables.

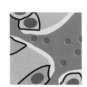

When you're planning a diet to reduce cancer risk, aim to do the following:

Include 5 to 9 servings of fruits and vegetables, aiming for a wide variety. Include dark green leafy varieties, deep yellow/orange varieties, cruciferous vegetables (cabbage, cauliflower, etc.), citrus fruits, berries, and other types daily.

Maintain a desirable body weight.

Bulk up your diet with lots of different types of high fiber foods (see Chapter 15).

Eat a varied diet—go for that third step in nutrient density you read about in Chapter 11; try to include at least 10 different foods (15 is even better) today, and a different 10 (or 15) tomorrow.

Cut your fat intake to a maximum of 30% of calories, eventually working your way down to 20%.

Limit alcohol consumption (if you drink alcohol at all).

Limit the amount of salt-cured, smoked, and nitrite-cured foods (which are associated with a greater risk of cancer of the esophagus and stomach when eaten in excessive quantities). When you do eat them, try to combine them with a food high in vitamin C, which may offer some protection.

How Food Protects You Against Cancer

As part of a healthy lifestyle, an abundantly nutritious, varied diet can protect you against many types of cancer. Here are a few examples of cancer-fighting foods and how they might work.

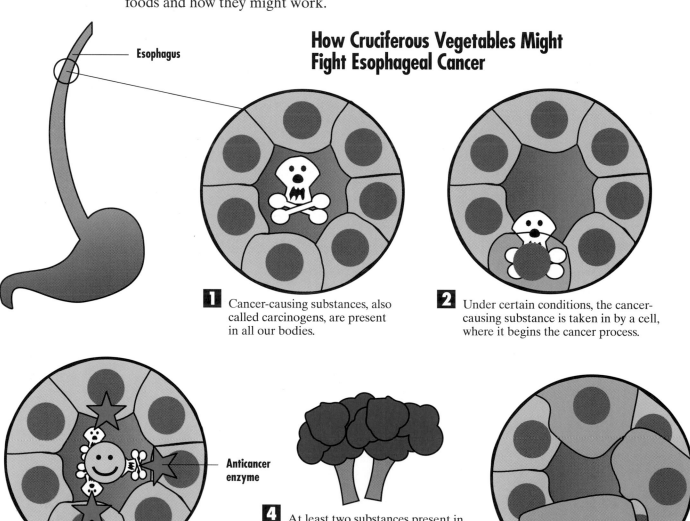

How Cruciferous Vegetables Might Fight Esophageal Cancer

Esophagus

1 Cancer-causing substances, also called carcinogens, are present in all our bodies.

2 Under certain conditions, the cancer-causing substance is taken in by a cell, where it begins the cancer process.

Anticancer enzyme

4 At least two substances present in the cruciferous vegetables (such as broccoli, brussels sprouts, and cabbage), called isothiocyanate (or sulforaphane) and indoles, somehow prevent normal cells from ever taking in carcinogens.

5 Isothiocyanates and indoles may do this by producing anticancer enzymes that either repel the carcinogen or detoxify it.

3 If unchecked, the cancer cell grows and invades other cells, producing a tumor.

How Soybeans May Decrease Risk of Breast Cancer

Scientists know that Asian women, whose diets are high in soybeans, have a lower incidence of breast cancer—some five to eight times lower. Although scientists aren't exactly sure how a substance in soybeans, isoflavone, decreases breast cancer risk, they think it does so by the actions below.

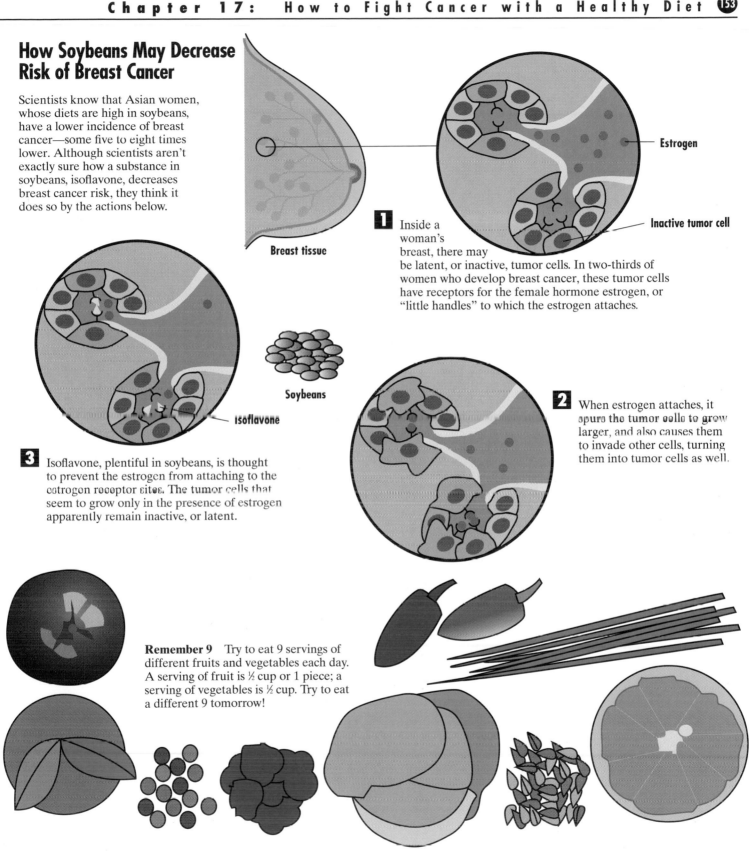

Breast tissue

Estrogen

Inactive tumor cell

1 Inside a woman's breast, there may be latent, or inactive, tumor cells. In two-thirds of women who develop breast cancer, these tumor cells have receptors for the female hormone estrogen, or "little handles" to which the estrogen attaches.

Soybeans

Isoflavone

2 When estrogen attaches, it spurs the tumor cells to grow larger, and also causes them to invade other cells, turning them into tumor cells as well.

3 Isoflavone, plentiful in soybeans, is thought to prevent the estrogen from attaching to the estrogen receptor sites. The tumor cells that seem to grow only in the presence of estrogen apparently remain inactive, or latent.

Remember 9   Try to eat 9 servings of different fruits and vegetables each day. A serving of fruit is ½ cup or 1 piece; a serving of vegetables is ½ cup. Try to eat a different 9 tomorrow!

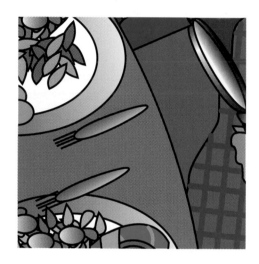

You Still Have Questions

WE HOPE BY now that you've realized that *from the food you eat* you can get all the nutrients you need to fuel your body and prevent many diseases. We hope you've even decided to toss your vitamin and mineral tablets and simply buy more healthy foods (ladies, hang on to your calcium and iron supplements).

No doubt, though, you still have some remaining questions about the foods you eat and the beverages you drink. In these final pages, you'll find some answers.

Is caffeine bad for me?   Caffeine, found in coffee, tea, cola beverages, chocolate, and some over-the-counter medications, is indeed a mild central nervous system stimulant. That means it can make you more alert, and at higher doses it can cause a rapid heart rate, jitteriness, irritability, and insomnia (especially when consumed too late in the day). At excessive doses, it can cause headaches, anxiety, and depression.

But for most people, consuming moderate amounts of caffeine-containing substances (the equivalent of 1 to 3 cups of coffee daily) causes no trouble. Extensive research has failed to turn up any link between caffeine and heart disease, including high blood pressure. Recently, the U.S. Surgeon General's Report, *Nutrition and Health*, reported that any rise in blood pressure due to caffeine consumption is less than the elevation produced by climbing stairs and other normal daily activities. In people who experience irregular heartbeats, or palpitations, caffeine can cause *more* irregular heartbeats; such people are well-advised to avoid caffeine.

Although you might have read at one time that caffeine causes pancreatic cancer, that original study was subsequently withdrawn; there's been no further evidence. Extensive research, in fact, has failed to turn up any link between caffeine and cancer in general.

Women with fibrocystic disease are frequently told to eliminate caffeine from their diet to reduce this often painful, but harmless, condition. However, many experts doubt this association. The best advice: If caffeine worsens *your* symptoms of fibrocystic disease, then reduce the amount you consume or eliminate it.

Although the results are inconclusive, a woman who wishes to become or is pregnant should probably cut down or eliminate caffeine intake, for two reasons. First, some (inconclusive) research suggests that caffeine may impair fertility. In addition, some animal research provides compelling evidence that caffeine may cause birth defects. Although human studies are not as convincing, a lingering doubt remains. Because of this, the U.S. Food and Drug Administration advises pregnant women to moderate caffeine intake.

Can I be a vegetarian and still get all the nutrients I need? It depends on how you craft your vegetarian diet.

There are three basic types of vegetarians: *Vegans* eat only foods of plant origin (they don't consume any dairy products, such as milk, nor do they consume eggs); *fruitarians* eat primarily fruits, nuts, honey, and vegetable oils; *lacto-vegetarians* eat dairy products and plant foods; and *lacto-ovo-vegetarians* consume eggs in addition to dairy products and plant foods.

As we've said throughout this book, the best way to get all essential nutrients is to eat a wide variety of foods, varying your menu meal by meal and day to day. This cardinal rule of good eating makes it easy to see why the more you restrict your diet, the more difficult it is to get essential nutrients. Most lacto-ovo-vegetarians and lacto-vegetarians get all critical nutrients—with two exceptions: They might come up short on B-12 and iron. Vegans have to keep a special eye on calcium, vitamin D, zinc, and vitamin B-6, as well as B-12 and iron (this is of special concern for vegetarian children and adolescents, who may have an especially difficult time getting essential nutrients and calories to meet growth demands). Vegetarians who consume no animal products need to supplement their diet with a reliable source of vitamin B12. Most experts recommend that vegetarians choose a variety of foods to assure nutritional adequacy. For example, fruitarians cannot possibly eat a healthy diet; this highly restricted diet is simply not recommended.

All vegetarians have to be careful about an unexpected problem: excessive fat intake. Because they're not eating meat, many vegetarians mistakenly think their diet is naturally low in fat. But vegetarians include more nuts and nut butters (tahini, peanut butter, and so on) in their diet, and many recipes call for a considerable amount of oil. Watch the nuts, nut butters, and oil, and you'll avoid this trap.

Does beef on the market today still have that dangerous *E. coli* I've read about? *E.coli 0157:H7* will always be present on a small percentage of beef (unless food irradiation becomes more widespread). One of the newest germs to cause foodborne illness is a special strain of *E.coli*, which scientists call *E. coli 0157:H7*. *E. coli* is a family of bacteria that exists normally—and innocently—in the intestines of healthy people and animals. Recently, however, this not-so-innocent strain of *E. coli* has emerged and caused outbreaks of foodborne illness. Although it doesn't bother the animals in which it resides, it can cause serious, even fatal, illness in people who consume it.

Here's how the bacteria causes illness—and why you shouldn't worry. The primary source is improperly cooked ground beef. Please note: Food with this bacteria is not spoiled, nor is it "bad" beef. The food simply was not cooked properly. *E. coli* is normally present just on the surface of beef—even cooking a steak to medium rare will destroy that surface bacteria (that's why you don't hear about other beef causing this type of illness). Ground beef is problematic because when the meat is ground, those surface bacteria become distributed throughout the patty. Just ensure that the hamburger you eat is cooked until its interior is no longer pink, and you needn't worry.

Does the process of food irradiation make food radioactive? Absolutely not! Irradiation, in fact, is one of the best and safest ways to destroy harmful disease-causing organisms on food without changing its nutritional value. Irradiation, for example, could destroy *E. coli 0157:H7* on beef; kill insects or prevent them from reproducing, thereby reducing food losses; and delay mold growth in fresh fruits, thereby prolonging shelf life. The main reason this technology is not used more is that many people remain leery of it.

Here's what you should remember about food irradiation. It does not make food radioactive; the doses and energy levels of radiation approved for the treatment of foods simply do not have enough energy to induce radioactivity in food. Also, the process does not generate radioactive wastes; the process simply involves exposing food to a source of radiation. It does not create any new radioactive material.

Does sugar cause hyperactivity? Many parents and teachers wonder about this, especially on the day after Halloween when candy-overloaded children are particularly "wound up." But there's no evidence that sugar induces hyperactivity in children with no known history of hyperactivity or that it worsens hyperactivity in children so afflicted.

Do food additives cause cancer or health problems? Are they responsible for behavior problems in children? Fortunately, there is no evidence that food additives (substances added to color, preserve, and flavor foods) cause behavior problems in children or cause cancer or other health troubles. Food additives must undergo rigorous testing to ensure their safety. If there is any hint that a substance causes any health problems, it simply isn't allowed. Many experts, in fact, believe that some additives have been banned from use without adequate evidence. There may be the rare child (or adult) who doesn't tolerate one additive or another—but this is the exception rather than the rule.

Should I be concerned about pesticides in food, especially fruits and vegetables?
Above all else, remember that the dangers of not eating fruits and vegetables far out-weigh any risks from eating the minute quantities of pesticide residue that may remain on food—the U.S. Food and Drug Administration, the Centers for Disease Control and Prevention, and the American Cancer Society all agree with this advice. But most encouraging of all, extensive monitoring of food for pesticide residues reveals that there simply is no reason to be concerned. The FDA's continuous food monitoring program found that less than 1% of foods had pesticide residues exceeding allowed levels (the FDA sets limits for pesticide levels, which have at least a hundred-fold margin of safety built in). An astonishing 98% of government-tested food samples contain little or no residue at all. Even in the small percentage of foods exceeding allowed standards, you're protected by that margin of safety. If you eat so much as to erase that margin of safety, your chances of experiencing ill effects are somewhere in the range of one-in-a-million. Your risk of becoming ill from food poisoning—eating improperly cooked or spoiled food—is many times greater than your risk of becoming ill from pesticide residue.

It behooves everyone to wash fruits and vegetables well, using a scrub brush not only to wash off trace pesticides but also disease-causing organisms.

What is monosodium glutamate? Monosodium glutamate, or MSG, is a naturally occurring amino acid used to enhance the flavor of food. It doesn't actually have a flavor of its own, but when added to certain foods, it amplifies other flavors. Some people become very ill if they eat foods with MSG, suffering dizziness, headache, and burning sensations. Fortunately, the new food label (which became mandatory in 1994) requires that manufacturers specify that MSG is in a product, which helps sensitive people avoid it.

Is there any advantage to buying "organic" produce? None whatsoever. An apple is an apple, and you simply can't alter the basic vitamin or other nutritional content substantially by changing the way it's grown. Organic food producers' main claim is that their produce is free of pesticide residues—but they don't tell you that the organic fertilizer they used (often animal or even human waste from sewage treatment plants) may pose an even greater danger to your health.

How to Put It All Together

As you plan your feast, take some hints from Miles, Sherlock, and our gardener. Above all else, maximize variety—choosing at least 10–15 different foods daily—and minimize fat. Highlight grains, vegetables, and fruits, accenting them with a wide variety of meat, fish, and poultry. Also, eat foods you enjoy, a critical key to weight control.

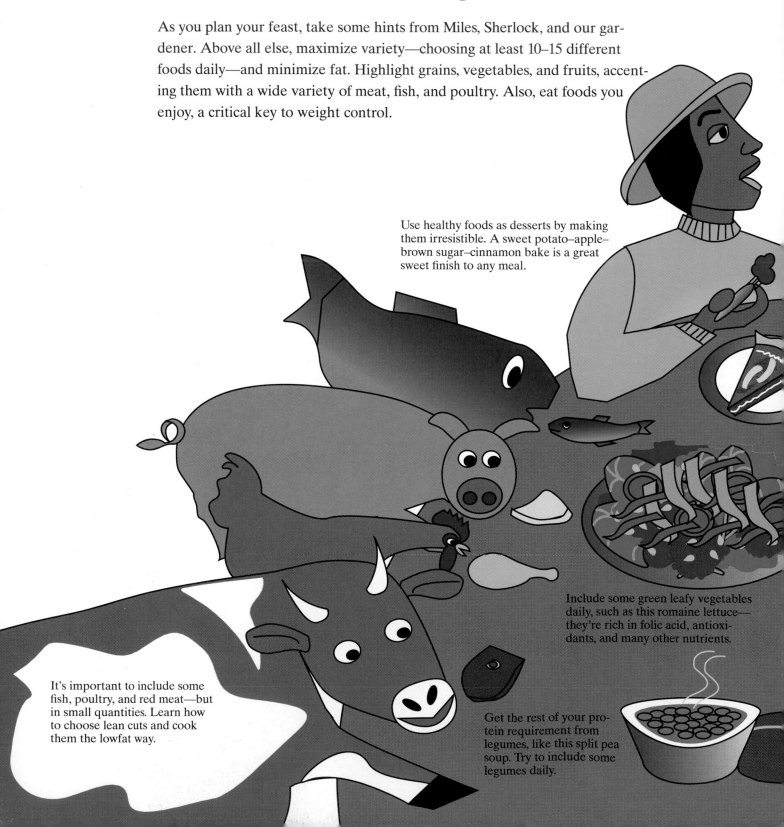

Use healthy foods as desserts by making them irresistible. A sweet potato–apple–brown sugar–cinnamon bake is a great sweet finish to any meal.

Include some green leafy vegetables daily, such as this romaine lettuce—they're rich in folic acid, antioxidants, and many other nutrients.

It's important to include some fish, poultry, and red meat—but in small quantities. Learn how to choose lean cuts and cook them the lowfat way.

Get the rest of your protein requirement from legumes, like this split pea soup. Try to include some legumes daily.

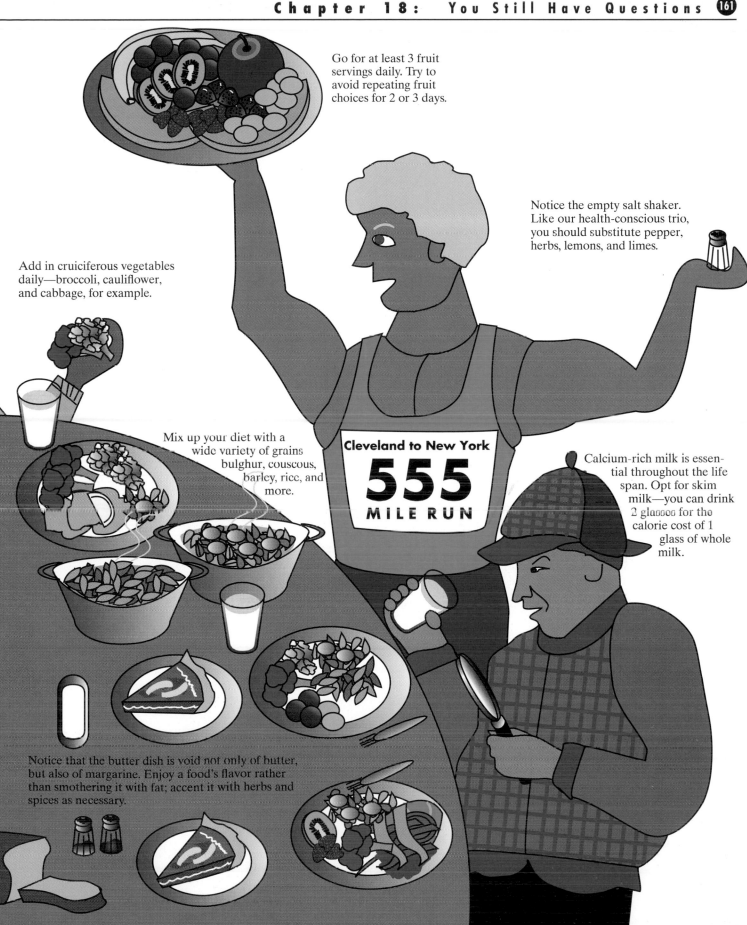

Go for at least 3 fruit servings daily. Try to avoid repeating fruit choices for 2 or 3 days.

Notice the empty salt shaker. Like our health-conscious trio, you should substitute pepper, herbs, lemons, and limes.

Add in cruiciferous vegetables daily—broccoli, cauliflower, and cabbage, for example.

Mix up your diet with a wide variety of grains bulghur, couscous, barley, rice, and more.

Cleveland to New York
555
MILE RUN

Calcium-rich milk is essential throughout the life span. Opt for skim milk—you can drink 2 glasses for the calorie cost of 1 glass of whole milk.

Notice that the butter dish is void not only of butter, but also of margarine. Enjoy a food's flavor rather than smothering it with fat; accent it with herbs and spices as necessary.

Critical Acclaim for *How Nutrition Works*

"Nutrition can be a complex science that seems far removed from what to eat for dinner tonight. *How Nutrition Works* translates the science of nutrition into food you should eat, in a readable, understandable way with clever illustrations and tips you can take to the grocery store—today!"

—Karen Miller-Kovach, M.S., R.D., Nutrition Consultant

"*How Nutrition Works* is written in a clear, easy-to-understand manner. The book is innovative in its approach, translating the theory of nutrition into practical terms. Napier explains how to formulate a healthy diet, always using foods readily available in grocery stores. She uses a groundbreaking approach to help the reader understand complex scientific information. This book belongs in the kitchen of every household!"

—Eric Mood, M.P.H., LL.D.
Associate Clinical Professor of Public Health (retired)
Yale University School of Medicine

"This book doesn't preach and it doesn't treat readers like bad children who subsist on cheeseburgers and fries. Instead, *How Nutrition Works* is a compendium of friendly, sensible advice from a professional who is clearly in the reader's corner. And why not? There's no rule that says celebrities should be the only ones with professional nutrition advisors."

—Patricia Thomas, Editor, *Harvard Health Letter*

A

albumin, 23

alcohol, drinking, 117

amino acid pool, 22

amino acids, 15–25

amino acid supplements, 18

angiotensin, 23

antioxidants, 147–148

   hall of fame, 69

   how they work, 68–69

   menus using, 68–69

   vitamins as, 65–69

appetite vs. hunger, 142

arteries, blocked, 113

ascorbic acid (vitamin C), 59, 65–69, 148, 150

atherosclerosis, 113

B

bad cholesterol, 29, 66, 123

balancing macronutrients, 35–43

beef. *See also* meat

   E. coli in, 156–157

   reference table, 40

beta-carotene, 49, 65, 69

biotin, 59

blood pressure

   controlling, 125–131

   and exercise, 127

   sodium and, 128–129

bone loss, 81–85

bones, vitamins and, 50

bradykinin, 23

breads

   high-fiber, 133

   reference table, 42

breast cancer, 153. *See also* cancer

bulk fiber, 116

B vitamins

   B-1 (thiamin), 58

   B-6 (pyroxidine), 58, 118

   B-3 (niacin), 58

   B-12 (cobalamin), 59, 118

   B-2 (riboflavin), 58

   and heart disease, 118

C

caffeine, 155–156

calcium, 81–85, 127, 129, 131, 148

   how the body uses, 84–85

   as iron inhibitor, 92

   and salt in the diet, 125

calcium supplements, 83

calories

   dividing between food categories, 38–39

   from fat, 29, 105, 109

   from fat vs. carbohydrate, 29

   getting nutrition from, 35, 38–39, 99–100, 102–103

   reference table of totals needed, 38

cancer
  and dietary fat, 149–150
  how fiber helps prevent, 138–139
  fighting with a healthy diet, 147–153
  fighting with vitamins, 50, 66
  and food additives, 157
  how food protects against, 152–153
carbohydrate calories vs. fat calories, 29
carbohydrates, 5–13
  complex, 5–9, 42, 133
  getting without excess fat, 42–43
  how the body burns, 12–13
  how nature makes, 10–11
  simple, 5–9
carotenoids, 49
cataracts, 69
categories of food, 35–39
cell membranes, building healthy, 32
cereal grains
  as complex carbohydrates, 8
  as high in fiber, 134–135
cheese reference table, 41
chicken reference table, 41
cholesterol, 27
  in the body, 120–121
  eating to lower, 113–123
  HDL (good), 114, 123
  LDL (bad), 29, 66, 114, 123
  and saturated fat, 115
chromium, 74
cobalamin (B-12), 59, 118

collagen, 23, 79
colon cancer, 134, 138–139
complementing proteins, 16, 25
complete proteins, 16
complex carbohydrates, 5–9, 42, 133
cooking oils
  comparison table of, 123
  monounsaturated, 29
  olive oil, 116
  polyunsaturated, 29
copper, 73, 78–79
corn syrup, 6–7
crackers reference table, 42
cruciferous vegetables, 152
cytochrome c oxidase, 78

D

daily value % (on food labels), 109
dessert reference table, 43
diastolic blood pressure, 125
dietary fat. *See* fat (dietary)
dieting, how to stop, 141–145
disaccharides, 5–6, 11

E

E. coli in beef, 156–157
elastin, 79
elderly, nutrient-deficient, 99
epithelium tissues, 49
esophageal cancer, 152. *See also* cancer

essential amino acids, 15–16, 21

essential fatty acids, 28, 32

exercise

   and lowering blood pressure, 127

   the many benefits of, 143

   and raising HDL cholesterol, 115

F

fat calories vs. carbohydrate calories, 29

fat (dietary), 27–33

   comparison of types of, 122–123

   daily calories from, 105

   getting carbohydrates without excess, 42–43

   getting protein without excess, 40–41

   how the body uses, 32–33

   meals with less, 110–111

   monounsaturated, 122–123

   polyunsaturated, 122

   and reducing cancer risk, 149–150

   reference table of suggested daily intake, 111

   saturated, 28, 108, 115, 122

   source foods, 30–31

fatty acids, 28

   body functions requiring, 32–33

   essential, 28

   trans fatty acids, 29

fat-soluble vitamins, 49–55

fiber, 148

   bulking up on, 135

   food with high fiber, 137

   getting enough, 133–139

   how it controls weight, 136

   and lowering cholesterol, 116–117

   and preventing cancer, 138–139

   types of, 133–134

fibrin, 23

fluoridated water, 73

fluoride, 72–73

folate, and heart disease, 118

folic acid (folacin), 57, 59, 148

food additives, 157

food categories, 35–39

   minerals in, 76–77

   and water-soluble vitamins, 60–61

food irradiation, 157

food labels, reading, 108–109

free radicals, 65, 68–69

fruitarians, 156

fruits, 7

   adding to the diet, 67

   as complex carbohydrates, 8

   eating more, 153

   juicing, 135

G

garlic, 116

globulin, 23

glucose, 5, 13

good cholesterol, 123

grains reference table, 41

grocery store walk throughs, 30–31, 36–37

H

HDL cholesterol, 114, 123

HDLs, 121

healthy and varied diet, 150, 160–161

heart disease, 113

    foods thought to prevent, 116–117

    vitamins to prevent, 118

heme iron, 91

hemoglobin, 91, 96

high-fiber breakfast cereal, 134–135

high-fiber foods, 133, 137

hunger vs. appetite, 142

hyperactivity and sugar, 157

hypertension, controlling, 125–131

I

incomplete proteins, 16

insoluble fiber, 133–134

iron, 91–97

    absorbing more, 94–95

    bodily needs for, 92–93

    a day's worth, 94–95

    how the body uses and reuses, 96–97

    leached from an iron pan, 93

    types of in foods, 91

iron enhancers, 92

iron inhibitors, 91–92

irradiation of food, 157

isoflavone, 153

J

juicing fruits and vegetables, 135

K

keratin, 23

L

lacto-ovo-vegetarians, 156

lacto-vegetarians, 156

LDL (bad) cholesterol, 29, 66, 114, 123

LDLs, 121

legumes

    as complex carbohydrates, 8

    reference table, 41

linoleic acid, 28

lipids, 27

lipoproteins, 120–121, 123

low-fat diet, devising, 105–111

lysine, 18

M

macronutrients, 1

magnesium, 72, 127, 129, 131

manganese, 74

meat. *See also* beef

    protein from, 18–19

    sodium in processed, 127, 130

menopause and bone loss, 84

metabolism and diet, 142

methionine, 18

micronutrients, 45

minerals, 46–47, 71–79

mineral supplements, 74

mitochondria, 78

monosaccharides, 5–6, 11

monosodium glutamate (MSG), 158

monounsaturated cooking oils, 29

monounsaturatcd fat, 122–123

muscle proteins, 16, 23

N

new food label, 106, 108–109, 126

niacin (B-3), 58

nonessential amino acids, 15–16, 21

nonhcme iron, 91

number of vs. type of calories, 3

nutritional supplements. *See* supplements

nutrition density, 99–100, 102–103

Nutrition Facts food label, 106, 108–109

nuts, 117

nyctalopia, 49

O

oat bran, 116–117

occluded arteries, 113

oils (cooking)

   comparison table of, 123

   monounsaturated, 29

   polyunsaturated, 29

olive oil, 116

omega-3 fatty acids, 123

organic produce, 158

osteoclasts, 55

osteoporosis, 81–85

oxalic acid, 83

oxidation, 65

P

pantothenic acid, 59

pasta refcrencc table, 42

pepsin, 23

peptides, 20

pesticides on food, 158

phosphorus, 73

phytochemicals, 148–149

pills. *See* supplements

polypeptides, 20–21

polysaccharides, 5, 11

polyunsaturated fat, 122

polyunsaturated oils, 29

pork reference table, 41

potassium, 127, 129, 131

potato reference table, 43

processed foods, sodium in, 127, 130

processed meats, sodium in, 127, 130

protein, 15–25

   animal sources of, 24

   complementing, 16, 25

   complete and incomplete, 16

a day's worth, 18, 24–25

getting without excess fat, 40–41

how the body uses, 22–23

how nature makes, 20–21

plant sources of, 25

protein deficiency, 16

psyllium, 116–117

pyroxidine (B-6), 58

R

Recommended Dietary Allowances
    (RDAs), 46

red blood cells, 91, 96–97

red meat. *See* beef; meat

red wine, 117

Reference Diet, 38–39

refined sugars, 6

retinol, 49

riboflavin (B-2), 58

rice reference table, 42

S

salts in the diet, 125–131

salt sensitivity, 125

salt substitutes, 130

satiety, 142

saturated fat, 28, 108, 115, 122

selenium, 73, 148

serving size (on food labels), 108

simple carbohydrates, 5–6, 9

snacks reference table, 43

sodium

    and blood pressure, 128–129

    forms of, 126

    limiting intake of, 125–126, 130

soluble fiber, 133–134

soybeans, 153

sparing protein, 17

starch, 5–6

sterol, 27

sucrose, 5

sugar, 5–6, 157

sun, vitamin D from, 53

supplements, 46–47

    amino acid, 18

    calcium, 83

    mineral, 74

    vitamin, 46–47

    vitamin D, 55

systolic blood pressure, 125

T

thiamin (B-1), 58

total fat (on food labels), 108

triglycerides, 28, 114–115, 122

turkey reference table, 41

V

varied and healthy diet, 150, 160–161

vegan diets, 156

vegetables

    adding to the diet, 67

    complex carbohydrates, 8

    cruciferous, 152

    eating more, 153

    juicing, 135

vegetarian diets, 156

vitamin A, 49–50, 52, 65, 67, 148

vitamin A precursors, 32

vitamin C, 59, 65–69, 148, 150

vitamin D, 50–51, 148

    taking with calcium, 83

    what the body does with, 54–55

vitamin D supplements, 55

vitamin E, 51, 53, 65–66, 68–69, 148

vitamin E supplements, 118

vitamin K, 51–52

vitamins, 46–47

    as antioxidants, 65–69

    fat-soluble, 49–55

    water-soluble, 57–63

W

walnuts, 117

water-soluble vitamins, 57–63

    how the body uses, 62–63

    in food categories, 60–61

wine, 117

Y

yo-yo dieting, 141

Z

zinc, 72

Introducing the Expanded Line of Lavishly Illustrated
"How It Works" Books from Ziff-Davis Press.

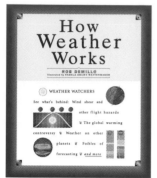

How Weather Works
ROB DEMILLO
Illustrated by PAMELA DRURY WATTENMAKER

● WEATHER WATCHERS

See what's behind: Wind shear and other flight hazards ☙ The global warming controversy ☙ Weather on other planets ☙ Foibles of forecasting ☙ *and more*

ISBN: 1-56276-228-1
Price: $19.95

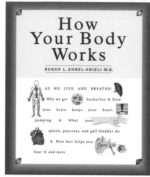

How Your Body Works
SUSAN L. ENGEL-ARIELI M.D.

AS WE LIVE AND BREATHE

Why we get ☙ backaches ☙ How your brain keeps your heart pumping ☙ What your spleen, pancreas, and gall bladder do ☙ How hair helps you hear ☙ and more

ISBN: 1-56276-231-1
Price: $19.95

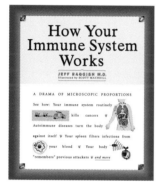

How Your Immune System Works
JEFF BAGGISH M.D.
Illustrated by SCOTT MACNEILL

A DRAMA OF MICROSCOPIC PROPORTIONS

See how: Your immune system routinely kills cancers ☙ Autoimmune diseases turn the body against itself ☙ Your spleen filters infections from your blood ☙ Your body "remembers" previous attackers ☙ *and more*

ISBN: 1-56276-233-8
Price: $19.95

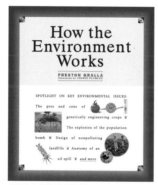

How the Environment Works
PRESTON GRALLA
Illustrated by CHERIE PLUMLEE

SPOTLIGHT ON KEY ENVIRONMENTAL ISSUES:

The pros and cons of genetically engineering crops ☙ The explosion of the population bomb ☙ Design of nonpolluting landfills ☙ Anatomy of an oil spill ☙ *and more*

ISBN: 1-56276-232-X
Price: $19.95

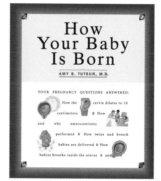

How Your Baby Is Born
AMY B. TUTEUR, M.D.

YOUR PREGNANCY QUESTIONS ANSWERED:

How the cervix dilates to 10 centimeters ☙ How and why amniocentesis performed ☙ How twins and breech babies are delivered ☙ How babies breathe inside the uterus ☙ *and more*

ISBN: 1-56276-239-7
Price: $19.95

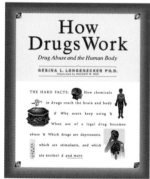

How Drugs Work
Drug Abuse and the Human Body
GESINA L. LONGENECKER PH.D.
Illustrated by NELSON W. HEE

THE HARD FACTS: How chemicals in drugs reach the brain and body ☙ Why users keep using ☙ When use of a legal drug becomes abuse ☙ Which drugs are depressants, which are stimulants, and which are neither ☙ *and more*

ISBN: 1-56276-241-9
Price: $19.95

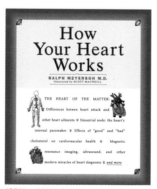

How Your Heart Works
RALPH MEYERSON M.D.
Illustrated by SCOTT MACNEILL

THE HEART OF THE MATTER:

Differences between heart attack and other heart ailments ☙ Sinoatrial node: the heart's internal pacemaker ☙ Effects of "good" and "bad" cholesterol on cardiovascular health ☙ Magnetic resonance imaging, ultrasound, and other modern miracles of heart diagnosis ☙ *and more*

ISBN: 1-56276-238-9
Price: $19.95

This fall, Ziff-Davis Press raises health and science books to an art form with an exciting expansion of the "How It Works" concept that sold over 800,000 copies in its first 18 months.

Why do people love "How it Works"? It's easy to see. Self-contained layouts place an entire topic before the reader's eyes all at once on a set of facing pages. Dramatic, full-color graphics invite them to explore at their own pace. It's a concept so simple, so natural, you'd think it has been done before. It hasn't. Not like this.

How did we pull this off? We auditioned hundreds of authors to find the chosen few who know their stuff and can put it in writing. Backing them up are consulting editors who are equally expert in their field and gifted illustrators who combine topic knowledge with a passion for presentation.

Who reads "How It Works"? Everyone who ever felt too intimidated to ask a doctor a question. Everyone who ever marveled at the miracle of childbirth. Everyone who ever lost a picnic to an unforecast hailstorm. In fact, just about everyone.

Watch for many more subjects in the months ahead!
Available at all fine bookstores, or by calling 1-800-688-0448, ext. 261.

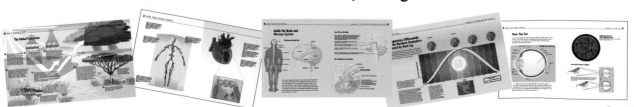

ZIFF-DAVIS
ZD
PRESS

© 1994 Ziff-Davis Press